THE
CALCIUM
CONNECTION

A Revolutionary Diet and Health Program to Reduce Hypertension, Prevent Osteoporosis, and Lower the Risk of Cancer

by
Dr. Cedric Garland
and
Dr. Frank Garland
with Ellen Thro and the assistance of
Eva Louise Garliano

A Fireside Book
Published by Simon & Schuster Inc.
New York   London   Toronto   Sydney   Tokyo

FIRESIDE
Simon & Schuster Building
Rockefeller Center
1230 Avenue of the Americas
New York, New York 10020

1   3   5   7   9   10   8   6   4   2   Pbk.

Library of Congress Cataloging in Publication Data

Garland, Cedric.
The calcium connection.
"A Fireside Book."
Reprint. Originally published: New York:
Putnam, c1988.
Bibliography: p.
Includes index.
1. Calcium in the body.   2. Vitamin D in human
nutrition.   3. High-calcium diet.   4. Cancer—
Prevention.   5. Hypertension—Prevention.   6. Osteo-
porosis—Prevention.   I. Garland, Frank Caldwell,
1950–   .   II. Title.
QP535.C2G37   1989   615'.2393   88-24365
ISBN 0-671-67192-8 Pbk.

ACKNOWLEDGMENTS

Many people have helped us with this book. Several gave enormous time and effort in assisting us. Edward D. Gorham, our friend and esteemed colleague, made such a wide range of contributions to the success of the book that it would require a catalog of activities to list and thank him for each.

There are several individuals who did not take part in writing the book, but whose research work, cited in the book, made many sections possible. Dr. Elizabeth Barrett-Connor of the Department of Community and Family Medicine of the University of California San Diego was a leading force behind one of the key scientific studies on which parts of this book are based. Dr. Michael H. Criqui of the same department arranged an important collaboration and contributed to these studies. Dr. Richard B. Shekelle of the Department of Epidemiology of the School of Public Health of the University of Texas Medical Center at Houston generously allowed use of data from a population he and his colleagues had carefully followed. We were then able to collaborate on a study which is described in this book. We greatly value the warm collegiality and spirit of scientific cooperation of these friends.

Our students have been a source of help and encouragement. Julia Lynn Vandenburgh assisted greatly during data collection and literature review on some of the studies cited in the book. Medical student Jeffrey Young, who completed a research project on urbanization and mortality rates from breast cancer with us, helped us to recognize and understand why air pollution and urban living are important factors in the risk of fatal breast cancer. Epidemiology student Eddie Ko Shaw helped with the studies reported in this book in a number of ways, particularly with respect to water supplies and air pollution.

A number of specialists across a range of fields generously shared their expertise. These included Wayne Hering, Dr. Jerome Namias, and Dr. Hans Panofsky of the University of California Scripps Institution of Oceanography, who advised on atmospheric optics and meteorological factors. Dr. James Pitts of the Statewide Air Pollution Research Center at the University of California at Riverside provided helpful information on the atmospheric chemistry of air pollution. Dr. George Mount of the National Oceanic and Atmospheric Administration in Boulder, Colorado, calculated the effect of sulfur dioxide on transmission of ultraviolet light, and Dr. Arlen Kruger of the National Aeronautical and Space Administration Goddard Space Flight Center provided satellite data from the TOMS instrument on the Nimbus 7 satellite that we used in determination of loss of ultraviolet light due to sulfur dioxide air pollution. Dr. Joseph Scotto of the National Cancer Institute provided detailed data on ultraviolet light.

The book would not exist if Sandra Dijkstra had not recognized the need for it and brought us together. We owe her major thanks. Mr. Roger Scholl, our editor, was both incisive and understanding. Numerous colleagues provided information of value, and we thank them for their help. The best qualities of the book are due to those who helped us, but responsibility for the contents is ours alone.

The late Dr. Abraham M. Lilienfeld of the Department of Epidemiology of the Johns Hopkins University School of Hygiene and Public Health had faith from the earliest days in our belief that ultraviolet light, vitamin D, and calcium play a role in risk of breast and intestinal cancers, and we are grateful for his encouragement to nurture the idea.

Finally, thanks are due to our families for endless patience and hope.

C.G.,   F.G.,   E.T.,   E.L.G.
La Jolla, California

This book is dedicated to Gene and Mary Viola
for their imagination and belief.

CONTENTS

Introduction

OUR CALCIUM AND VITAMIN D DISCOVERY

The Calcium Connection began as a result of our recent news-breaking discovery with colleagues that a diet rich in calcium and vitamin D can help to prevent intestinal cancer. The connections between calcium and osteoporosis, and calcium and high blood pressure have been previously described by other medical scientists. With our discovery of the link between certain types of cancer and calcium, however, we realized, as never before, the essential role calcium plays in our health.

In addition to the critical importance of calcium in the body, we realized that vitamin D plays an important and overlooked auxiliary role. Too often the calcium in the food we eat is unusable. Because of this, health-conscious people may think they are taking in enough calcium according to the various calcium charts and counters currently available, when they are not—because much of what they have taken in cannot be absorbed.

Vitamin D helps the body absorb calcium and plays a major role in the body's ability to use the calcium that is available. An awareness of the role that vitamin D plays in calcium absorption, as well as familiarity with natural calcium "robbers" (foods that bind calcium and make it unusable) will make an important difference in whether or not you get enough usable calcium daily. *The Calcium Connection* is the first book to bring together all these factors to fashion a complete calcium program that can be tailored to each individual's needs.

THE CALCIUM–CANCER LINK

It has been widely reported that calcium plays a role in osteoporosis and high blood pressure, but our research is the first to link a deficiency of calcium to cancer.

Our discoveries about calcium and vitamin D are grounded in exacting scientific facts—evidence that shows that the risks of breast and intestinal cancer in the United States and throughout the world vary according to geography. In the United States, generally the farther south people live, the lower the risks of breast and intestinal cancers. People in some northern U.S. cities have *three times* the risk of dying from these cancers as people in the south. There are even bigger differences in risk among other countries. The question, of course, is why?

Our investigation began on a summer afternoon in 1979. We were sitting in a lecture hall at the Johns Hopkins University, where Cedric was a member of the faculty and Frank a graduate student. We were viewing a presentation of maps of the United States showing the rates of various cancers for each of the 3,056 counties in the United States, information newly computed by Dr. T. J. Mason and his colleagues of the National Cancer Institute. On each map, the parts of the country with high rates were darkly colored, and areas with the lowest rates were white. Most of the maps showed a random, shotgunlike pattern of light and dark. But two maps—one of breast cancer and one of intestinal cancer—struck us with their startling geographic pattern. Although we didn't know it then, we were beginning to unravel an epidemiologic mystery.

It looked as if someone had drawn a heavy line along the thirty-seventh parallel—through the middle of California, and the tops of Arizona, New Mexico, Texas, Tennessee, and the Carolinas. Virtually all the places, with high mortality from breast and intestinal cancer were north of this line, whereas those with low mortality were south of it. The white low-cancer areas were far more frequent in the sun belt. For example, most of southern California and Arizona were white, as was New Mexico. The dark areas,with high mortality, were located in the northern half of the country, particularly in the northeast.

Cedric had a flash of inspiration. Could the rates for intestinal and breast cancer be connected somehow with sunlight? Our first step in answering the question was to try to eliminate other possible explanations for the geographic differences. One such possibility involved food. Both fiber-containing vegetables and red meat had been strongly suggested as influences in the occurrence of colon cancer—fiber as a food that helped to *prevent* the disease, and fat and red meat *increasing* its likelihood. Fat had been strongly suggested as a cause of breast cancer, as well. Perhaps eating patterns were different in various parts of the United States.

We obtained dietary consumption patterns for the nation from a survey conducted by the Department of Agriculture. The survey told us that food consumption is remarkably similar throughout the United States, including intake of fruits, vegetables, fats, and red meat. Supermarkets and fast-food restaurants have standardized American eating habits, so geographic differences in food consumption didn't explain the vast differences in intestinal and breast cancer rates across the country.

Our next step was to look at all evidence available to test the theory. We examined patterns of cancer death rates from around the world looking for clues about sunlight and other cancers. One of the first observations we made was that the death rates throughout the world for intestinal and breast cancer were much higher in big cities than in small cities and towns at the same latitude. We guessed that people in big cities at any latitude were deprived of vitamin D as adults due to air pollution and indoor urban lifestyles.

SUNLIGHT, VITAMIN D, AND CALCIUM

What was the significance of sunlight with regard to cancer rates? Sunlight reacts with cholesterol inside and on the surface of the skin to create vitamin D. Vitamin D helps the body absorb calcium (the correlation between calcium and cancer will be discussed in Chapter 1). Here's how it works:

Three hormones regulate calcium in the body; only one, vitamin D, is to some extent under our control. Vitamin D is the only vitamin that has both a dietary and nondietary source. It is present in a few foods, such as fortified milk and some kinds of fish, but what makes vitamin D so unique is that it's also produced when the skin is exposed to sunlight. Sunshine activates the cholesterol on the skin, creating provitamin-D. A reaction requiring body heat transforms this to vitamin D, which is transported to the liver and kidneys in sequence, where each adds a molecule to it. The final product is transported to the small intestine, where it directs the cells lining the intestine to produce a calcium-binding protein from a part of their DNA, or genetic material. This protein then lies in wait, ready to yank in any unsuspecting calcium coming through the intestine. Once hooked, the calcium is carried everywhere in the body it is needed, including the breast and the rest of the intestine. Without vitamin D, most of the calcium is cast off, completely unused.

Calcium is one of the great binders of nature: it causes cement to harden, blood to clot, bones to hold up. Every cell in the body uses it. It's needed for your nerves to fire, for your brain to function, and for your muscles to contract. Even your heart won't beat without calcium.

What is the relationship between calcium and cancer? Calcium maintains the organization of tissues. Tissues are groups of cells that do the body's work. Coordination among the cells in a tissue is maintained mostly by bridges, known as tight junctions, that bind the cells together physically and allow messages to be carried among them. The messages are carried by calcium atoms just like messages on a telephone line are carried by electrons.

Tight junctions—and communication between cells—disappear when calcium in the fluid around the cells drops. The tissues become disorganized. Competition among the cells for food and oxygen replaces the usual cooperation, and a process of rapid evolution at the cell level begins.

The result of this is that highly specialized, aggressive cells evolve that can command resources, invade other tissues, and kill other cells. This is cancer.

THE WESTERN ELECTRIC STUDY

In 1984, an opportunity arose to test the effects of dietary vitamin D and calcium on intestinal cancer in a group of 1,954 men. The men were employed by the Western Electric Company in a telephone assembly plant near Chicago. They were given dietary interviews during 1957–58, and were followed-up carefully for occurrence of heart disease and cancer by a distinguished group of scientists, including Drs. Richard Shekelle, Arthur Rossof, Oglesby Paul, and Jeremiah Stamler.

Our friends and colleagues Drs. Michael Criqui and Elizabeth L. Barrett-Connor of the University of California San Diego Department of Community and Family Medicine met Dr. Shekelle at an educational conference on heart disease epidemiology. Both Dr. Criqui and Dr. Barrett-Connor mentioned our theory to Dr. Shekelle, and suggested that it could be tested using the study that Shekelle's group in Chicago had begun years before. Dr. Shekelle agreed and we began the analyses.

The study, which we coauthored with Drs. Barrett-Connor, Criqui, Shekelle, and his colleagues Drs. Rossof and Paul, was published in *The Lancet* on February 9, 1985. Dietary histories were collected at the beginning of the study, *before* any disease occurred. The participants cooperated faithfully during the next nineteen years, and all but three of the men remained in the study to the end.

Intestinal cancer takes about twenty years to develop. We knew that patterns of intestinal cancer according to foods eaten would be evident because twenty years had passed since the study began. Diet histories for the study had been collected by nutritionists using plastic models to precisely measure the quantities of food eaten during the month before the interviews. The averages of each participant's two histories, one year apart, became the basis of the study. Information on the foods the men ate and their intake of vitamins and other nutrients was calculated and stored for later analysis. At the end of the period, forty-nine of the men had developed colon or rectal cancer and 1,372 men were free of cancer (the rest died of other causes).

We found that men who developed intestinal cancer were a little heavier than those who did not, but they consumed slightly fewer calories than those free of cancer. A typical American high-fat intake (43 percent of the men's calories were from fat) was present in both groups. The two groups ate virtually identical amounts of animal and vegetable protein and carbohydrates. There were no significant differences in intake of saturated or unsaturated fats, dietary cholesterol, minerals (except calcium), and most vitamins. The intake of alcohol differed slightly: heavier drinkers had a slightly higher risk of intestinal cancer.

Much to our excitement, our findings showed that the men who developed intestinal cancer differed from those who did not in only two respects—they ate far fewer foods containing vitamin D and calcium. Men who took in calcium and vitamin D equivalent to four glasses of nonfat milk per day had only about *one third* the risk of intestinal cancer.

The men in the lowest intake group of vitamin D took in about

60 International Units (IU) per day, which is less vitamin D than found in an ordinary glass of nonfat vitamin D-fortified milk (100 IU); whereas the men in the highest intake group took in an average of 336 IU per day, or the amount of vitamin D in three-and-one-third glasses. The men who had the lowest intake of vitamin D developed about twice as much intestinal cancer as those who had the highest intake (Figure 1).

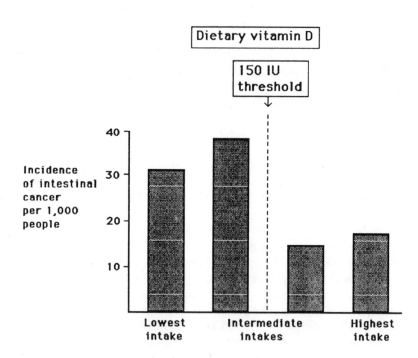

Figure 1. *Dietary vitamin D intake and incidence of intestinal cancer in 1,954 Western Electric men during 19 years. (Source: Garland C, Shekelle RB, Barrett-Connor E, Criqui MH, Rossof AH, Paul O. Dietary vitamin D and calcium and risk of colorectal cancer: a 19-year prospective study in men.* Lancet 1985;1:307-9.)

There was a threshold effect at 150 IU vitamin D—the amount in one-and-one-half glasses of milk. The threshold effect means there was no additional decrease in risk of intestinal cancer for men who consumed more than 150 IU of vitamin D per day.

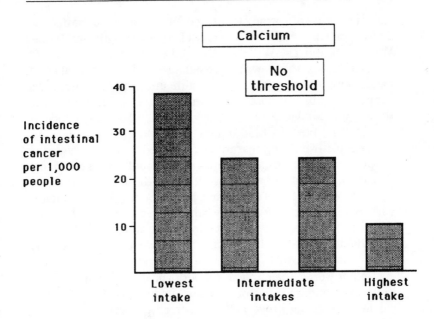

Figure 2. Calcium intake and incidence of intestinal cancer in 1,954 Western Electric men during 19 years (Source: Garland C, Shekelle RB, Barrett-Connor E, Criqui MH, Rossof AH, Paul O. Dietary vitamin D and calcium and risk of colorectal cancer: a 19-year prospective study in men. Lancet 1985;1:307-9.)

Figure 2 shows the incidence of intestinal cancer according to intake of calcium. Men who took in the lowest amount of calcium (on average about 625 milligrams per day, or the amount of calcium in two glasses of milk) had more than three times as much intestinal cancer as men who had the highest intake (1,200 or more milligrams per day, or the amount of calcium in four glasses of milk). There was no threshold for the benefit of calcium. This means that we do not know the upper limit of protection that calcium can provide. The more calcium the men took in, the lower the risk they had.

THE LABORATORY TEST

Cedric was invited to the Memorial Sloan-Kettering Cancer Center in New York to present these findings, where the results were warmly received.

Dr. Martin Lipkin and Harold Newmark of Sloan-Kettering were studying New Yorkers who were at high risk of intestinal cancer because of a strong family tendency to develop the disease. They were pursuing work Newmark had begun with Dr. Michael Wargovich and Dr. W. R. Bruce at the University of Toronto, Canada. Lipkin and Newmark designed a study to see what effect calcium might have on the tissue of the intestinal tracts of these people. They used a dose of calcium that was about the same as the one we found to be associated with the lowest risk of cancer in our *Lancet* study of Chicago men.

The Sloan-Kettering researchers reported that these high-risk people, before taking calcium, had an unusually high rate of cell division in the intestine. During the test, these people took calcium at a dose of 1,250 milligrams per day in the form of calcium carbonate. After two or three months of the dietary supplements, their intestinal cells stopped dividing at the abnormally high rate and adopted a rate of cell division typical of people at ordinary risk of intestinal cancer.

In other words, the clinical test performed at Memorial Sloan-Kettering Cancer Center verified our predictions of the effect of calcium on cancer growth at the microscopic level.

A CURIOUS EXCEPTION

There was still one exception to our general findings about the connection between sunlight, calcium, and cancer. That exception was one that had been drummed into us by Dr. Abraham Lilienfeld at Johns Hopkins. "Breast cancer is almost nonexistent in Japanese women," he would say, "and we have no good explanation. Perhaps someone in this room will discover why."

Breast and intestinal cancers are most prevalent in places far from the equator. Most residents of Japan live between 33 and 45 degrees north of the equator, a region with only moderate sunlight. The amount of sunlight reaching Japan is associated almost everywhere else in the world with high rates of breast and intestinal cancer. But the rate of these cancers in Japan is very low — about 5 per 100,000. By comparison, other areas at the same latitude, such as San Francisco and Connecticut, have rates more than five times as high.

We felt that Japan was the odd case, the final telling clue. The meaning of the clue was first discovered two hundred years before, although until our research no one connected the finding with breast cancer. It involved immunity to a disease in Japan that was then causing severely malformed bones in English children. The disease, rickets, was so common in London that it was called the English Disease. It first appeared when the English began burning coal on a grand scale in London as early as 1600. As increasing amounts of ash from the coal rose into the atmosphere, the pollution became so bad that it blocked London's sunlight. Before long, everything in the city was coated with gray soot—buildings, trees, even butterflies. In fact, the dark gray butterflies that were appearing everywhere were not just coated with soot—the butterflies were actually emerging from the cocoon dark gray, an early sign of natural selection at work. Light-colored butterflies were quickly seen by birds against the soot-covered buildings and were eaten. Darker butterflies were blending into the background. In a few centuries the whole population of butterflies had turned gray.

With urban coal burning and industrialization came bowed legs, knock-knees, and deformities of the chests and pelvises of infants and children. The disease became so troublesome in England that one scientist—a medical explorer—traveled to Japan, where the disease was rare, to find out why. What he found was a population virtually free of rickets, and people who ate a diet loaded with fish.

This aspect of the Japanese diet, which still includes huge amounts of fish, suggested a cure for rickets to that early epidemiologist. It now suggests to us the reason why rates of breast and colon cancer were so low in Japan. Fish is loaded with vitamin D. Although the Japanese do not receive a great deal of sunlight, their *diet* provides the vitamin D their bodies need to help absorb calcium, and prevent breast and colon cancers. This was the missing link, the exception, that confirmed our theories about vitamin D, sunshine, calcium, and cancer.

The connection between calcium and cancer had been confirmed. It was but one more way in which we found calcium to be so essential to health. It was at this point that we decided to consolidate our research and the research of so many before us on calcium and its effects, and bring our findings to the general public. More important, given how crucial calcium is to health, we conducted further research to come up with a complete nutritional program to:

1. determine how much calcium and vitamin D *you* need, and

2. offer a dietary progam to increase the amount of *usable* calcium in your diet.

By following *The Calcium Connection* program, you can ensure that you are getting enough calcium—usable calcium—to help safeguard against osteoporosis, high blood pressure, and cancer. To discover more about the role calcium plays in the body, and how you can increase your calcium intake, read on.

PART I
CALCIUM'S
ROLE
IN THE
BODY

1

Calcium and Your Body

The human body cannot manufacture calcium. We obtain calcium by eating or drinking foods that contain calcium. On a typical day, the average person takes in about one fortieth of an ounce of calcium, roughly the weight of a small feather (700 milligrams). Unfortunately, usually only 15–35 percent of the calcium we eat is absorbed by the body, depending upon a person's age, sex, vitamin D availability, and the presence of other foods that block calcium absorption.

What happens to the calcium that is absorbed? Your body will first allocate the calcium to your blood. If the calcium level in your blood is adequate, it will be shunted quickly to the extracellular fluid around your cells. The extracellular fluid surrounds each cell in your body and gives it the essentials that the cell needs for survival.

Calcium from the extracellular fluid around the cells that make bone will be put to work. You are always making new bone. The process, called remodeling, allows the body to develop new and powerful bones throughout a person's lifetime. The ability to strengthen and develop new bone cells is particularly important for those who are physically active and during pregnancy.

A 40-year-old man taking in an average amount of calcium for his age (700 milligrams) might absorb only 245 milligrams per day. At the same time, his body will lose 100 milligrams of the absorbed calcium in solid waste, 150 milligrams in urine, and 20 milligrams in sweat each day. He will have lost 270 milligrams, but only absorbed 245, leaving him with a daily loss of 25 milligrams.

After a period ranging from minutes to hours, some of the calcium that is absorbed will be used to form a crystal called apatite in the bones throughout the body. It will move fastest to bones which specialize in storing calcium for fast access. These bones, called trabecular bones, are the body's equivalent of a 24-hour market, open day and night to meet unexpected needs.

Some of the calcium that is absorbed goes to the kidneys, which excrete about 150 milligrams per day. The kidneys conserve calcium; only one one-hundredth of the amount of calcium that enters them is excreted under normal circumstances, although drinking lots of coffee, for example, can change this ratio, causing the kidneys to excrete much more calcium than they would normally.

CALCIUM'S JOB IN YOUR BODY

Calcium is used in two ways in your body. The first is for communication. The cells in your body talk constantly, using a special chemical code. They routinely communicate information necessary for your tissues to function properly.

Calcium is vital to that communication between cells. Cells exchange information through tiny bridges between them, called calcium channels. Most calcium channels are located in structures called communicating junctions. Cells transmit various kinds of messages, and we hypothesize that the most important of these is a "vote" to an adjacent cell on whether to divide.

A normal cell in tissue called epithelium—the cells that make up the inside layer of your intestine, your skin, and which line the ducts of a woman's breasts—collects "votes" on whether to divide from adjacent cells apparently using a calcium channel.

HOW CALCIUM GOVERNS CELL DIVISION

Your body can be seen in a sense as a giant cooperative venture with billions of cells working toward a common objective, your health.

Many of the most important tissues in your body have an outermost layer that is only one cell thick. This is true of the cells lining the intestine, the cells in the lungs that exchange oxygen and carbon dioxide with the air we breathe, and the cells lining the inside of most of our internal organs. In the case of the small intestine, for example, a single layer of cells is devoted to absorbing nutrients.

What does this mean in terms of calcium and cell communication? Cells exchange information or communicate by sending calcium ions from one cell to a neighboring cell via a communicating junction. When contact between cells is cut off for some reason, we believe that cells interpret this as the loss of a neighboring cell. The apparent loss of nearby cells seems to stimulate the proliferation of cells that make new epithelium.

This is the secret of the calcium connection. Calcium carries a vital message between the cells that keeps them from dividing unnecessarily. When calcium in the fluid bathing the cells is very low, the communication system is disconnected. The cells can't receive signals from adjacent cells. If enough time passes without receiving signals from other cells, the cells that make new epithelium will divide. If the two cells produced do not receive signals from other cells, they too will divide. If the four cells produced by their division do not receive signals via calcium channels from other cells, they too will divide, producing eight cells, and so on.

Before long, there will be several generations of new cells, each generation doubling the size of the previous generation. If these cells do not continue to receive growth-blocking signals via calcium channels from adjacent cells, they will continue to proliferate in a chain reaction. Soon the cells will form a pileup, and take on peculiar shapes and sizes. When the pileup is large, the condition is called hyperplasia.

Hyperplasia may be physical evidence of the breakdown in communication among cells. In the intestine, it appears long before cancer is present. The usual scenario of a breakdown in communication in the cells of the intestine may be for the cells to pile up until they form a polyp, which is an unusual extension of the lining of the intestine into the lumen, or opening, where the food passes through. The cells are limited in how far they can expand back into the tissue, so eventually there isn't anywhere for them to go except out into the lumen.

If you look at polyps under a microscope you will see that many are disorganized tissues. Most polyps don't start out as cancer, but rather seem to be a result of the body's attempt to deal with epithelial cells that are needlessly dividing due to a deficiency of calcium in the fluid bathing them.

How does proper cell communication prevent uncontrolled cell division? We believe signals sent through a communicating junction to an adjacent cell informs it that another cell is nearby. Signals such as these sent from the surface of the cell are used by the cell nucleus, the specialized central headquarters, to make a decision about the need to reproduce.

If the signals coming to the cell membrane are constant, adjacent cells are considered to be present. If the signal from one surface of the cell stops coming in, it means that the adjacent cell is no longer present. Perhaps it had been washed away, as often happens in tissues such as the intestine. Or the cell might have died, shrinking slightly and leaving space.

CALCIUM, CELL DIVISION, AND CANCER

This function of calcium has opened up a new window on the way cancer works. It may be the missing piece in a puzzle that has bedeviled scientists since the earliest days of cancer research.

Cancer, we think, happens in three phases: decoupling, initiation, and promotion. It is the first phase, which we call decoupling, where calcium has the greatest effect.

Decoupling

Decoupling is the process of cells splitting apart from one another. It happens when the amount of calcium in the extracellular fluid is low. It is due to loss of tight junctions that bind cells of the intestine, breast, and some other tissues together. As we discussed above, cells in many tissues will divide unless they receive a signal from neighboring cells. If that signal is blocked, as with a piece of plastic film between the cells, then cells on both sides of the film begin to divide.

Most cells in your body are constantly taking "votes" on the question of whether or not to divide. Calcium allows the "votes" to be communicated. Calcium passes easily from cell to cell, like electrons in an electrical wire, but only when the cells are in close contact. If for any reason, the close contact between cells is interrupted, it would be as if you had cut an important wire in an electrical circuit. The signal cannot be transmitted, and the cells that make new epithelium will begin to proliferate.

When cells lose communication and begin to divide on their own, the tissue becomes disorganized and the cells begin to pile up. This chaotic mitosis or cell division, that results in large crowds of cells, is called hyperplasia. If the cells are unusual shapes or are especially disorganized, it is called dysplasia. It isn't cancer, however—it often disappears spontaneously without a trace. Decoupling lays the groundwork for hyperplasia, which may precede the next stage in the formation of cancer, initiation.

Initiation

We think three of the primary requirements for cancer are decoupling, induced genetic variation and rapid turnover of cells. Radiation or toxic chemicals can produce variation by attacking the DNA in the cells, causing mutations. Most of the mutated cells will die but a few will thrive. Those that thrive are better able to get food and oxygen than normal cells, and therefore better able to reproduce.

If the generator of variation continues to act—if, for example, X-rays are continually applied or chemical carcinogens are continuously present—more variation will occur. New mutations will arise in each generation of transformed cells. Again, most will die but those that survive will do so because they have an advantage in getting food and oxygen. These cells in turn will thrive and reproduce. Those that reproduce most rapidly are the most successful. If this process continues over many generations, a generation of highly aggressive, rapidly reproducing, mutated cells will come into being. These cells become potent competitors for food and oxygen at the expense of normal cells. In many cases they lose their fine structure and even some of their genes. These are cancer cells.

If the generator of variation is removed, such as removing the carcinogen, or eliminating the radiation, the evolutionary process may be arrested before a new generation of cancer cells evolves. This is probably what happens, for example, when a person quits smoking. The predominant carcinogen in tobacco smoke is benzo-alpha-pyrene. Take it away and evolution of the cells toward cancer is usually arrested.

Sometimes the rescue may come too late. If the cancer cells have evolved sufficiently already, then taking away the generator of variation, or tobacco smoke, will do little good. The die has been cast. This is why quitting smoking late in life doesn't always prevent cancer.

Promotion

The third stage of cancer is proliferation of the highly evolved cancer cells. A cancer can be *promoted* by a chemical that is not a cause of variation. There are many chemicals, such as the hormone estrogen, that do not appear to initiate cancer cells, but which can stimulate them to grow. This is very practical information since it tells us we can arrest or retard the growth of cancers if we take away any promoters present. The rate of spread of breast cancer can be reduced dramatically in many women, for example, by eliminating the promoter estrogen. This can be done with a medicine known as tamoxifen, which is an estrogen blocker. Without the promoter, the cancer tissue slows its rate of reproduction. Unfortunately, it doesn't stop reproduction completely, so eliminating promoters does not cure cancer. But it can extend life.

HOW CALCIUM PREVENTS INTESTINAL CANCER

Calcium seems to prevent intestinal cancer in the decoupling phase of the disease.

When calcium levels drop in the fluid that bathes the cells, the tight junctions between the cells disappear. The reason they vanish is unknown, but their disappearance seems to be a self-protective mechanism intended to tide the cells over until the calcium level in the fluid bathing them rises.

It has an unfortunate side effect. It cuts off close contact with nearby cells. Cells can function normally without communication with other cells, at least for short periods of time. Eventually, though, in the absence of communication from other cells, the cells will divide. On the other hand, if calcium levels remain normal, cells will not divide unnecessarily, and the evolution toward cancer that is enhanced by abnormally rapid cell division will be slowed. A sufficient intake of calcium slows the evolution of normal cells toward cancer and can help to *prevent* it.

CALCIUM AND STRUCTURE

The second major role of calcium in the body is to provide structure. There are only a few elements in the world that are used routinely to provide structure for plants and animals. Almost all rigid structures of plants and animals contain calcium. Each cell in your body, with a few exceptions, has a skeleton, called a cytoskeleton, that keeps the cell together. These cell skeletons differ in degrees of rigidity, but in places where they must be very rigid they include crystals of calcium. The reasons for this are that calcium is strong, easily dissolvable, and transportable.

YOUR BONES

The same qualities that make calcium so expedient as a skeleton for the cells—its ability to be dissolved readily and moved from place to place—make it essential for strong bones as well. The disease osteoporosis, in fact, occurs because calcium is easily dissolvable and transportable. A more complete discussion of osteoporosis occurs in Chapter 3.

How are bones formed? In the months preceding birth, collagen, a tough substance used by the body where flexible strength is needed, forms a net where bone will be created. Calcium in the fetus is then carried from the placenta to this net, where the calcium crystals are neatly caught from one edge of the developing bone to the other. In the months and years that follow, more calcium is added to the bone structure, giving the bone strength.

Calcium is essential to the body at the cellular level, as a structural support and as a means of communication between cells, and in the formation and endurance of bones as well. Because of its importance throughout the body in a variety of functions, a sufficient calcium intake is crucial to health and fitness.

2

Calcium and Cancer

BREAST CANCER

Breast cancer is the most frequent cancer in women, and the most deadly. More women die of breast cancer than any other form of cancer. The incidence rate has been increasing steadily throughout the world. There are 130,000 new diagnoses and more than 40,000 deaths from breast cancer in the United States each year. We believe most of these deaths can be prevented.

The risk of breast cancer is highest in areas that receive low levels of sunlight (Figure 1). Because of this we studied the effects of sunlight on mortality rates of breast cancer in the United States.

The U.S. National Oceanic and Atmospheric Administration reports on sunlight striking the ground at a series of points throughout the country. With medical student Jeffrey Young, we located twenty-nine major cities and fifty-five rural areas where both data on sunlight and mortality rates were available. The data were specific for size of the population, age, and race.

With the help of fellow epidemiologist and friend Edward Gorham, we constructed a graph of the average daily sunlight versus the rate of fatal breast cancer for the major U.S. cities (Figure 2, page 32).

As we expected, the *more* sunlight a city received, the *less* the rate of fatal breast cancer. As you can see, the lowest rates were in

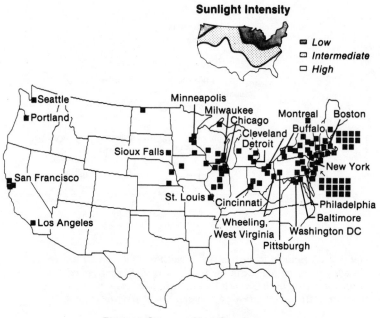

Breast Cancer Hot Spots

Figure 1. Breast cancer hot spots and sunlight intensity. Source: *National Cancer Institute.*

Honolulu, Phoenix, Albuquerque, Las Vegas, and El Paso. These cities received the highest amounts of sunlight of any cities in the United States (all in excess of 500 calories per square centimeter of land area per day).

The highest rates were in New York, Washington D.C., Chicago, Cleveland, and Boston. These are all cities that received much less sunlight (250–365 calories per square centimeter per day).

You will notice that New York, Washington D.C., Cleveland, Columbus, Los Angeles, and San Diego are all well above the line. They all have more breast cancer than expected based on average sunlight level alone. This points to an important factor in the

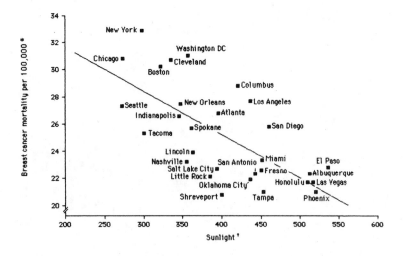

Figure 2. As sunlight levels increase, incidence of fatal breast cancer drops. Mortality rates are highest in the relatively sunlight-deprived cities of the northeast, lowest in the sunbelt and Hawaii. Sources: *National Cancer Institute, National Oceanic and Atmospheric Administration.*

sunlight equation: air pollution. These cities *all* suffer from some form of air pollution. Certain types of air pollution selectively block out a part of the range of ultraviolet light known as UV-B, the part of the sunlight spectrum (295–310 nanometers) that creates vitamin D in the skin and that causes sunburn. The result is that it is hard to get enough vitamin D from the sun in cities with significant air pollution.

The worst blockers of ultraviolet light among ordinary air pollution are sulfur dioxide and its atmospheric aerosols. This is the air pollution that results from burning coal with high sulfur content in commercial power plants and industries. Much of this coal is burned for cheap electric power in the Midwest and the Ohio and Tennessee valleys. Winds carry the thousands of tons of sulfur dioxide to the Northeastern part of the country, where it remains to block ultraviolet light and create aerosol compounds that reflect ultraviolet light back into space (Figure 3). Aerosols are suspensions of fine solid or liquid particles in air.

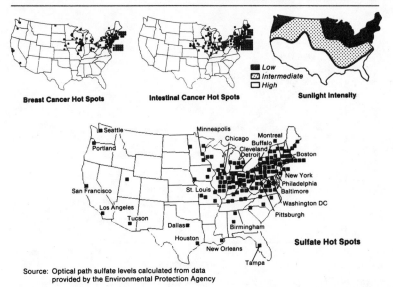

Breast Cancer Hot Spots

Intestinal Cancer Hot Spots

■ Low
▨ Intermediate
☐ High

Sunlight Intensity

Sulfate Hot Spots

Source: Optical path sulfate levels calculated from data
provided by the Environmental Protection Agency

Figure 3. Mortality from breast and intestinal cancers is highest in areas with high concentrations of airborne sulfate particles, sulfate "hot spots." Sources: Ambient concentrations of sulfur dioxide in the optical path were calculated from data provided by the Environmental Protection Agency and other reporting sources.

Less effective in removing ultraviolet light, but still of importance, is the air pollution found primarily in the southwestern part of the country, smog. Smog occurs when sunlight reacts with the exhaust from cars and pollutants from commercial power plants and industries (particularly nitrogen oxides) depleting ultraviolet light before it reaches the ground.

When we recently uncovered evidence of the powerful blocking effect of sulfur dioxide at the wavelength needed to make vitamin D, we added this factor to our analyses. When we did this, cities that were once above the diagonal prediction line (Figure 2) moved closer to a recomputed diagonal line (Figure 4, page 34). With these factors it is possible to explain 72 percent of the geographic variation in the occurrence of fatal breast cancer in the United States.

The impact of air pollution in major cities is magnified by urban lifestyles. Seventy-five percent of Americans live in cities, and urban dwellers spend the majority of their lives indoors. On week-

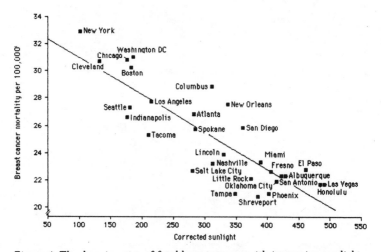

Figure 4. The drop in rates of fatal breast cancer with increasing sunlight becomes clearer when the measure of sunlight is adjusted ("corrected") for air pollution from sulfur dioxide and ozone. Los Angeles, New York, and several other cities with serious air pollution have moved closer to the diagonal line (compare with Figure 2) suggesting that sunlight is a better predictor of mortality rates when adjusted for the pollutants that block ultraviolet light. Sources: *Calculated from data provided by the National Cancer Institute and the National Oceanic and Atmospheric Administration.*

days, most people's brief exposure to the sun on the way to and from work occurs when little UV-B from the sun is present.

Urban architecture also cuts our exposure to sunlight. The concrete canyons between the skyscrapers of Manhattan receive only tiny amounts of sunlight, blocking 95 percent of sunlight on the street below. Even a row of ten-story buildings, small by Manhattan's standards, will delete virtually all sunlight from a city's streets. This may help explain why Manhattan has the highest rate of fatal breast cancer on the planet. No other location in the United States even comes close. There are other factors to consider as well, such as the relocation of women with breast cancer to Manhattan for medical care. Nonetheless, deprivation of light undoubtedly plays a major role in the city's astronomical breast cancer rate.

Seattle, on the other hand, is below the line (Figure 2). This means it has a lower rate of fatal breast cancer than would be expected from its sunlight rating alone. The reason? The sunlight that strikes the ground in Seattle contains virtually all of its UV-B and can create vitamin D in the skin. In Seattle, strong winds and a low level of sulfur dioxide pollution keep the sunshine full of ultraviolet light.

Most of the variation in rates of fatal breast cancer among the major cities of the United States can be explained solely on the basis of differences in sunlight and sulfur dioxide pollution. This is also true in small cities, towns, and rural areas. The skin produces more vitamin D in sunny places and people are protected by it because they absorb more calcium.

While sunlight is the clue that showed us why the risk of breast cancer varies from region to region, we don't advise that you spend more time in the sun, as overexposure to UV-B is a major cause of skin cancer. Instead, we recommend that you follow the dietary guidelines for *The Calcium Connection* diet presented later in the book.

A DEEPER LOOK AT THE RELATIONSHIP BETWEEN AIR POLLUTION, LIGHT, AND CANCER

Take a careful look again at Figure 3. The figure shows sulfur dioxide (SO_2) air pollution, and the inserts show maps of hot spots of fatal breast cancer, intestinal cancer, and sunlight intensity.

When you first glance at the maps you can see the relationship. The reason is that the areas with high sulfur dioxide pollution levels also have high rates of breast and intestinal cancer.

Sulfur dioxide pollution, in particular, selectively filters out the part of ultraviolet light that creates vitamin D. It is the lack of vitamin D that results in the increased incidence of fatal breast and intestinal cancer.

After a few days in the air, sulfur dioxide converts to aerosols of sulfuric acid and ammonium sulfate, and remains for days to weeks strongly reflecting UV-B back into space. The people living in areas with high pollution from sulfur dioxide and its aerosols cannot produce vitamin D in their skin except during two or three months a year. Like many Americans, they get so little vitamin D from their diet and sunlight that they are seriously deficient in it.

Take another look at Figure 3, and you will have an idea how much sulfur dioxide is present in the atmosphere where you live. The more sulfur dioxide, the less ultraviolet light, and the more you will need to supplement your diet with vitamin D and calcium, up to the amounts we recommend on page 82 . Sulfur compounds in the atmosphere play a major role in predicting the risk of vitamin D deficiency diseases.

Seattle, again, has low pollution from sulfur dioxide and its aerosols and also low rates of breast and intestinal cancer, considering its latitude. Westerly winds may blow Seattle's sulfur dioxide away from the city before most aerosols form. New York has the highest levels of sulfur dioxide aerosol pollution. The rate of fatal breast cancer in New York is nearly double that of Seattle, and the rate of fatal intestinal cancer in New York is also much higher.

Aerosols created by sulfur dioxide create a diamondlike sheen that reflects the sun's brilliant ultraviolet light back to space, over New York and the northeast, leaving a shadow nearly devoid of the ultraviolet wavelength that creates vitamin D. Add to these particles of soot and dirt in the atmosphere from industry, and you have a curtain of darkness covering the northeastern United States and parts of Canada. The sulfur dioxide and nitrogen oxides in the atmosphere also cause acid rain and acid fog.

New Hampshire and Maine are hundreds of miles from major U.S. industrial centers, and the rural lifestyle outside the main cities in these areas would normally be expected to be healthy. The reverse is true. Beautiful rural New Hampshire and Maine, two of the most pastoral places in the United States, have higher rates of breast cancer than 46 other states, including the most teeming, heavily industrialized states. The rate is shockingly high in all of New York State, too—and the rate in the province of Quebec is higher than in any other part of Canada. The same is true for death rates from intestinal cancer. We believe these high cancer death rates are due primarily to the curtain of darkness from sulfur dioxide and its aerosols carried east by winds from power and industrial plants in midwestern America.

Worse, when breast and intestinal cancers strike in these regions, they are more likely to kill than in the sunny Southwest or in the clear-skied Pacific Northwest.

OZONE

Most of the ultraviolet light coming from the sun, about 99 percent, is filtered out by the Hartley Band of ozone, which is thickest about fifteen miles high. This band has existed for millions of years and protects us from dangerously high levels of ultraviolet light. Ozone concentrations drop off at five miles above the surface, and increase again at ground level, due to local air pollution.

A key example of ground level ozone pollution occurs in Los Angeles, where ozone levels become very high during the morning and afternoon rush hours. The photochemical reaction that produces ozone removes large portions of ultraviolet light, making Los Angeles sunlight deficient in the energy needed to produce vitamin D on days with high photochemical activity.

FISH, VITAMIN D, AND CANCER

Japan is at about the same latitude as San Francisco and receives about the same amount of sunlight, but as we discussed in the introduction, the rates of breast cancer are astronomical in San Francisco and very low in Japan. The reason for this, we believe, is the enormous amount of fish consumed daily in Japan, a food rich in vitamin D. Japanese have for centuries consumed six times the U.S.R.D.A. (U.S. recommended daily allowance) of vitamin D, or 1,200 IU. Very few people in the United States consume anywhere close to this amount.

Women who migrate from Japan to California have a radical increase in rates of fatal breast cancer. The rate in one area of Japan is 5 per 100,000 women; it rises to 57 in Japanese women who move to the United States. The reason for this is that the food the women eat changes dramatically with the move—Japanese women who have moved to California from Japan and who have taken on a U.S. diet consume one twentieth as much vitamin D as their relatives in Japan. Perhaps it's no surprise that Japanese women here have a higher incidence of breast cancer.

Many fish that are popular in Japan contain very high amounts of vitamin D. Salmon, a favored item, contains 500 or more IU of vitamin D per 3.5-ounce serving. A popular sushi bar specialty, Anago (eel), is the richest natural source of vitamin D in the world. A 3.5-ounce portion contains 5,000 IU of vitamin D.

The typical American woman consumes only a fifth to a tenth of the vitamin D she needs. Women from the United States, England, Scotland, Ireland, Canada, and New Zealand are at extremely high risk of fatal breast cancer. These are areas of relatively little ultraviolet light and extremely low intake of dietary vitamin D. In the Caribbean, Central America, or Africa, by contrast, where bright light is abundant, women have extremely low rates of breast cancer.

THE BABY BONUS

Women who have had children in parts of the world where vitamin D levels are high have a lower risk of breast cancer than childless women in the same areas. During pregnancy, vitamin D receptors appear in the tissues of the breast. These are molecules that help the breasts absorb vitamin D. The breasts in turn absorb more calcium. The purpose is to produce milk. The high level of vitamin D present in the breast during pregnancy and the absorption of calcium which it stimulates seem to cut the risk of the first stage of cancer. The benefit appears thirty to thirty-five years later as a flat blip in the climb of cancer incidence rates with age. We call this blip the *pregnancy plateau.*

Epidemiological studies of women in Japan, where intake of vitamin D is high, show a strong pregnancy plateau for breast cancer. Countries that have intermediate levels of vitamin D tend to have less evident plateaus and intermediate levels of protection associated with having babies. Countries such as the United States, Canada, and most of Europe, however, where vitamin D levels are low, show virtually no pregnancy plateau.

FAT AND CANCER

Contrary to widespread opinion, fat does not directly cause breast cancer. A number of years ago, researchers observed an apparent correlation between fat consumption in various countries and risk of breast cancer. But a recent long-term study of more than 89,000 nurses by Dr. Walter Willett and his colleagues of Harvard University, showed that the risk of breast cancer is unrelated to intake of fat in the usual U.S. dietary range (30–40 percent of total calories).

Dietary fat can bind calcium, however, making it less absorbable. We believe that persons who have a diet very high in fat may become deficient in absorbable calcium. Because of fat's ability to bind calcium, women with a high-fat and low-calcium diet could be at even higher risk of breast cancer than women who have only a diet low in calcium. We recommend that women cut fat intake to 20 percent of total calories to assure adequate calcium absorption. This level of fat intake will also reduce risk of heart disease.

INTESTINAL CANCER

The three leading causes of cancer death in the United States are lung, intestinal, and breast cancers. Ninety-nine percent of intestinal cancer is cancer of the colon (86 percent) and rectum (13 percent); the remaining 1 percent is cancer of the small intestine. You've just learned how to minimize your chance of getting breast cancer. If you're a male, there is no need to worry about getting breast cancer (only 400 men are diagnosed with it each year in the United States). The best answer to preventing lung cancer has been long established by epidemiologists—avoid smoking tobacco. By following the guidelines in *The Calcium Connection*, you may be able to cut your risk of intestinal cancer by two thirds, as well.

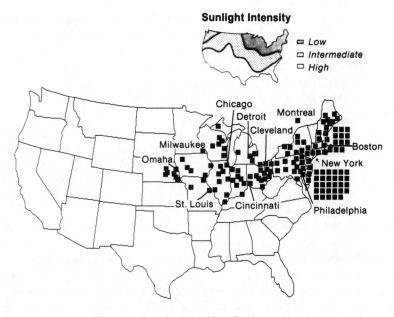

Intestinal Cancer Hot Spots

Figure 5. Fatal intestinal cancer, like breast cancer, hits hardest in areas with the least sunlight. This map shows counties with significantly high rates of cancer of the large intestine (colon). Counties with low sunlight levels (upper right) are the most affected. Sources: National Cancer Institute, National Oceanic and Atmospheric Administration.

As with breast cancer, the rates of intestinal cancer are significantly higher north of the dividing line than south of it. Within the high-rate area there are "hot spots," places where the rate is even higher. The leading cities in intestinal cancer hot spots in the continental United States are shown in Figure 5. The hot spots are based on reports of death rates for white females from the National Cancer Institute (NCI). Hot spots for intestinal cancer in men are virtually identical to those for women and therefore are not shown. Each hot spot has a mortality rate from cancer of the large intestine that is significantly higher than the U.S. average for white females. The rates have been adjusted by the NCI for age differences among cities, so the rate is not explained by the differences in the ages of the people who live there. Nor is it due to differences in race among the areas, since these maps show rates only for whites (maps for other races are available in publications of the NCI).

The small map inset on Figure 5 shows sunlight levels. The areas marked in solid black, including New York, Chicago, Boston, Philadelphia, New Haven, Pittsburgh, and Cleveland, receive the least sunlight of any of the 29 major cities, less than 365 calories per square centimeter per day. Montreal, Canada, receives 300 calories. All hot spots for intestinal cancer are in or near the low-sunlight zone.

There are no hot spots in the high-sunlight zone. This zone has many areas, shown as open boxes, where rates are significantly *lower* than the U.S. average. These include most counties in California's sunny San Joaquin Valley; Tucson and Phoenix, Arizona; Albuquerque, New Mexico; El Paso, Texas; and Miami, Jacksonville, Tampa, and Orlando, Florida.

The world over, intestinal cancer predominates in areas with little sunlight, either from weather or air pollution. The highest-risk areas in the world are: Manhattan; Birmingham, England; most of Germany; Connecticut; Warsaw, Poland; New Zealand; Denmark; Sweden; Leningrad; Moscow; and Montreal. The lowest risk places are: Ibadan, Nigeria; Dakar, Senegal; Honduras; Nicaragua; Chile; Sicily; and Japan. All high-risk areas receive less than 400 calories per day of sunlight per square centimeter of ground. All low-risk areas except Japan (whose people consume large amounts of dietary vitamin D) receive more.

HOW MUCH CALCIUM AND VITAMIN D IS ENOUGH?

The point behind all these studies is to show that the amount of sunlight, and therefore vitamin D, a person receives, varies according to geography and local conditions. People who receive a great deal of sunlight need *less* dietary vitamin D, because their bodies produce more vitamin D from the sun than people from low-UV-B areas. People in the north and in heavily polluted regions need *more* calcium and vitamin D because of the lack of sufficient vitamin D producing sunlight. The amount of calcium and vitamin D a person needs, therefore, varies.

The present recommended daily intake of vitamin D in most countries is 200 to 400 IU per day, which is the amount in two to four eight-ounce glasses of fortified milk. Similar amounts of vitamin D are available from ordinary servings of salmon or other kinds of fish, as shown later in the book under *The Calcium Connection* diet. You can find the amount of calcium and vitamin D you need from the charts listed in Chapter 8 of the book.

We don't recommend increasing the amount of sunlight you receive by exposing yourself for longer periods of time to direct sunlight. People who live in northern climates are usually not well adapted to strong sunlight, and run a considerable chance of developing skin cancer due to overexposure. For this reason, we suggest moderate or little intentional direct exposure to the sun, particularly from 10 A.M. to 2 P.M. The same wavelength of light that stimulates production of vitamin D in the skin, UV-B, increases the risk of skin cancer.

3

Calcium and Osteoporosis

As we discussed earlier in Chapter 1, your body cannot make calcium. The only way your body can obtain it is by eating or drinking foods that contain calcium. As we explained, your body needs calcium for a variety of reasons, particularly on the cellular level. If it does not obtain enough calcium from the foods you eat, your body's first tendency is to sacrifice calcium from its only reservoir—your bones—to provide calcium for those functions for which it is even more crucial. Ninety-nine percent of the calcium in the human body is stored in bones. When calcium in other parts of the body runs critically short, calcium from the bones is dissolved and carried away to those parts of the body that need it more. If the body goes for a long period of time with a calcium deficit, the bones can become extremely porous and brittle, resulting in brittle-bone disease, or osteoporosis.

The loss of calcium from the bones starts with the hip bones, the heads of the large leg bones, and the vertebrae, or spinal bones, which are the bones where calcium is stored for rapid access in time of need. People who have a calcium deficient diet may sacrifice small amounts of calcium from their bones for years without knowing it, until the bones break.

Keeping your bones strong and healthy is a lifelong proposition. Osteoporosis is not something you can overcome simply by ingesting more calcium after the fact. You cannot make up for years of calcium depletion in the bones by overloading your diet with calcium. The key to preventing osteoporosis is making sure that your body receives a sufficient amount of calcium day after day. You need to start a proper calcium program *today,* whether you are eighteen or eighty. We will tell you how to set up a proper calcium program in the chapters that follow.

CALCIUM DEFICIENCY

In order for calcium to be usable to your body, it must be absorbable. Most of the calcium your body takes in is not absorbed. Therefore it is important to distinguish between calcium and *usable* calcium—calcium that can be used by your body. If you are an adult, you will need to take in 800 to 1,200 milligrams of calcium per day (see chart on pages 82–83) for your body to absorb enough calcium to prevent osteoporosis, as well as other diseases resulting from an insufficiency of calcium.

Most adult women in the United States and many men lose calcium every day of their lives. Three quarters of women sixty and older consume less than 725 milligrams of calcium per day. We feel that 800 to 1,200 milligrams per day is needed, depending on your age, sex, and where you live, for most people to cut risk of the calcium deficiency diseases that become apparent in adulthood: osteoporosis, hypertension, and certain cancers. Currently 85 percent of women and the majority of men take in less calcium than they need.

The 800 to 1,200 milligram intake of calcium per day recommended for most people is in the context of the program outlined in this book, including intake of eight to twelve glasses of water a day, restriction of foods containing oxalates and excess salt, which lower calcium absorption, exercise, consultation with a physician or nutritionist, and other measures. Excessive intake of salt, especially intake of above 5 grams per day, increases urinary loss of calcium; high intakes of oxalate may increase risk of kidney stones in some persons.

Intake of calcium by men is nearly as poor as by women. Most men take in only 700 milligrams per day. Only a small portion take in the levels we recommend.

The amounts of calcium you need are high because the body absorbs so little. Our diet and lifestyle conspire to keep a typical urban adult from absorbing 65 to 85 percent of the calcium consumed.

Once you have absorbed calcium, your body can send it where it is needed. If you happen to absorb more than you need on a particular day, you will excrete more than usual to balance the high intake. In any event, your body has had a chance to get all the calcium you need. If you do *not* absorb enough calcium, your body will pay the price.

VITAMIN D DEFICIENCY

If you take in calcium, but there is too little vitamin D in your body, your body will not be able to absorb most of the calcium. Absorption of calcium is controlled by vitamin D.

When you are very young, your skin can produce vitamin D easily, but as you get older it cannot. Your skin produces half as much vitamin D at age sixty as at age ten, according to a recent study by Drs. J. MacLaughlin and M. Holick of Tufts University School of Medicine in Boston.

Your ability to absorb vitamin D from the food you eat also decreases with age, so it is especially important to take in your diet the suggested amounts of vitamin D recommended in *The Calcium Connection* for the area of the United States in which you live, and your age. A complete profile of your needs can be determined from the information in Chapter 7.

OSTEOPOROSIS

If your bones weigh too little for your size, you have low bone mass. If your bone mass is extremely low for your body size, or you have had a fracture due to low bone mass, you are considered to have osteoporosis. The bones have lost so much calcium that they become fragile, brittle, and susceptible to fractures. Osteoporosis increases the chances that one or more of your bones will someday break, perhaps during some minor traumatic event. The bones that usually break are the head of the femur (the bone from your hip to your knee) and the vertebrae, or spinal bones.

Contrary to popular thought, your bones are continuously broken down and rebuilt in your body. Bone dissolvers, or osteoclasts, are constantly tearing bone calcium and protein apart, while cellular building crews, or osteoblasts, work to build it back up. Some bones are entirely rebuilt or remodeled every five years, some faster.

Nevertheless, although the cells that make up bones are constantly active, bones are *not* at the top of the list in terms of the body's priorities for calcium. Instead, bones are at the bottom of the list. The calcium needs in the body, in terms of priority, are as follows:

Blood	Pancreas
Heart	Kidney
Brain	Liver
Intestine	Skin
Stomach	Bones

Because of this, it is hard to get the calcium that *is* absorbed to your bones. The bones are always at the end of the line when the body allocates calcium.

The problem is made worse because your intestines, if you are like most American adults, will not absorb most of the calcium you take in.

The epidemiology of osteoporosis can best be told by studies of the two harmful effects of the disease: fractures of the hip and fractures of the vertebrae. Most "hip" fractures are actually fractures of the head of the femur. Not all fractures of the head of the femur or vertebrae are due to osteoporosis, but many are.

There are big differences between countries in the incidence of hip fractures (see Figure 1, page 46). The United States is the world leader in hip fractures for men and women. The differences are not due to differences in age between the populations, because age differences have been taken into account. These results tell us that hip fractures aren't a part of the human condition. If they were, the incidence would be the same everywhere.

In fact, a woman living in Yugoslavia is only one sixth as likely to fracture a hip as a white woman in the United States. This is unlikely to be due solely to a genetic difference. Dietary deficiencies or environmental factors, such as a deficiency of light, lead to differences in the amount of vitamin D produced in the body, and, we believe, to increased risk of hip fractures.

A recent study in Yugoslavia illustrated the effect of diet. There are two similar towns in Yugoslavia that differ in an important way: intake of calcium. The towns aren't far apart and they share a rural Yugoslavian culture and way of life. But calcium intake in

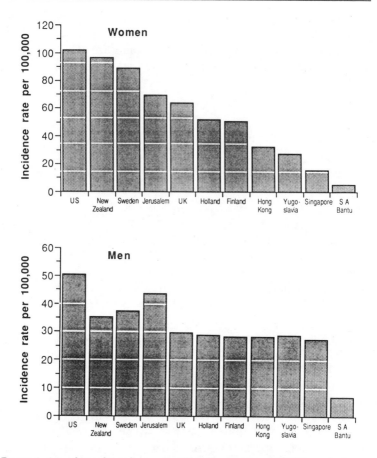

Figure 1. Age-adjusted incidence rate of hip fracture per 100,000 people, by location. Source: *Drawn from data provided in: Cummings SR, Kelsey JL, Nevitt MC, O'Dowd KJ. Epidemiology of osteoporosis and osteoporotic fractures.* Epidemiologic Reviews *1985; 7: 178–208.*

one city is much higher than in the other. The women and men who have lived in the high-calcium town have had only *half* the incidence of hip fractures as those in the low-calcium town (see Figure 2).

The scientists who studied these villages, Dr. V. Matkovic and a group of colleagues, published their results in the *American Journal of Clinical Nutrition.* Studies of bone mass were performed in the two towns and it was found that there was a difference in bone mass that was constant from the earliest age studied to the oldest.

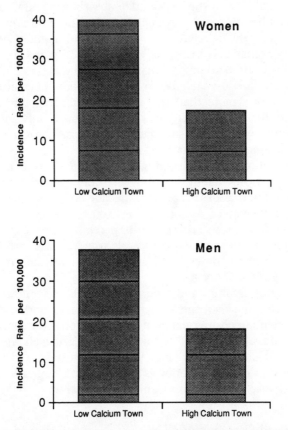

Figure 2. Risk of hip fractures in two Yugoslavian towns. Source: *Matkovic V, Kostial K, Simonovic I, et al. Bone status and fracture rates in two regions of Yugoslavia.* American Journal of Clinical Nutrition *1979; 32: 540–549.*

This suggests that the effect of absorbed calcium is lifelong. Calcium is needed to form bone. The sooner a calcium-rich diet is started, the better.

Calcium's Role in the Prevention of Osteoporosis

There are several factors that play a part in the development of osteoporosis. These include being white, female, slender, tall, sedentary, having low estrogen levels, smoking cigarettes, and having a high coffee intake. One reason a woman's bones may become fragile is that she has eaten or absorbed too little calcium throughout her life, gradually depleting the calcium in her bones to make up for the deficiency. According to government surveys, American women take in an average of 490 milligrams of calcium a day. This is 10 to 60 milligrams less than the 500 to 550 milligrams of calcium lost each day. When the amount of calcium lost is even slightly more than the amount taken in, bone loss is inevitable. Since 490 milligrams is the *average* daily intake of adult women, we can estimate that about *half* of American women are *losing bone throughout their adult lives.*

The condition is like a dripping faucet—the amounts involved are small, but they add up. You may lose only a few milligrams of bone a day, but this loss over several decades will leave you with a substantially reduced skeleton when you reach your sixties or seventies. If you lose 30 percent to 40 percent of your bone mass, your spinal column will gradually collapse. You will lose height and may develop "dowager's hump," a skeletal deformity for which there is no cure.

The role of calcium and vitamin D in the prevention of osteoporosis has not been entirely defined, but it is clear that women should remain in positive calcium balance throughout their lives. They should take in more calcium than they lose each and every day. The question of how much calcium you need and how to overcome a calcium deficiency is discussed in Chapter 8, in Part II of the book, The Calcium Connection program.

Exercise and Osteoporosis

Calcium and vitamin D will not increase the calcium content of bone without exercise. It is important that you adopt an exercise program as well as increase your calcium intake. Exercise makes bones work, strengthens them, even helps to remodel them. The activities of many women and men do not involve sufficient activity in hip and leg bones. Jobs that minimize use of the lower body, such as sitting at a desk, which many people do for years during their working lives, must be counterbalanced with vigorous activity. A regular program of weight-bearing exercise is essential.

A walking program will provide a starting point, but everyone ultimately should work toward a program of aerobic exercises, which provides structural benefits. Low- or nonimpact aerobics put healthful force on the bones of the legs and hips, which are weak points for the development of fractures later in life, without unduly stressing the joints.

Other forms of exercise are less effective. Doubles tennis, for example, does not provide enough mobilization of the long muscles over a sustained period of time to encourage much increased bone mass, and the staccato action of court sports can injure bones and tendons.

Swimming, while it is beneficial to the cardiovascular system and does not put undue pressure on the joints, does not create the necessary weight-bearing loads on the bones of the legs and hips to increase bone mass.

The Plague of Osteoporosis

It is estimated that by the year 2000, 40 percent of Americans will live to be eighty-five years old. This means we're going to be facing even more osteoporosis in the future.

Again, osteoporosis currently affects fifteen to twenty million people in the United States, and each year it will cause about 1.3 million fractures. Unless there is a sharp reversal in trends, 32 percent of elderly women and 17 percent of elderly men will suffer a hip fracture due to osteoporosis. The dark shadows cast by these predictions are based on statistical estimates published by the Consensus Conference on Osteoporosis of the National Institutes of Health, which appeared in the *Journal of the American Medical Association* in 1984.

Currently, nearly one third of the women residents of nursing homes are there because of fractures, and 85 percent of these are fractures of the hip. The fractures often follow some minor trauma that would normally not cause a broken hip. But because these women aged sixty and older have such fragile bones, a minor fall, or even stepping off a curb awkwardly, can result in a broken hip. These women, though, may not be aware that they have the crippling disease until the first fracture.

The consequences are serious. This is because a broken hip often requires a period of immobilization, and immobilization can be deadly. Extensive time in bed can sometimes result in pneumonia or the development of blood clots, either of which can be fatal; a third of women will die within a year of an osteoporotic hip fracture.

Estrogen

Estrogen also plays a role in the prevention of osteoporosis. Like vitamin D, it enhances the absorption rate of calcium in the intestine, and helps keep the bones from getting smaller. The reason why it has such an effect is not completely known. Because estrogen is beneficial, it is often prescribed to women suffering from osteoporosis. Although we would like to minimize the use of medication, women with osteoporosis, especially if they are beyond menopause, may need estrogen to prevent further bone loss and possible fractures. Before menopause, women's natural estrogen levels provide protection. Estrogen stimulates the absorption of calcium by the intestine and also seems to have its own effect in helping bones maintain their mass and strength.

The use of estrogen has certain risks. Cancer of the endometrium (part of the uterus) appears to be increased by use of estrogen, and the incidence of blood clots may be slightly higher in some women who receive the hormone. This is counterbalanced by a lower rate of heart disease in women taking supplementary estrogens. We understand the fear many women have of endometrial cancer. But women past the menopause are at least ten times more likely to die from heart disease than from endometrial cancer. The benefits of estrogen in minimizing the harm of osteoporosis may outweigh its risks. Of course, women who have had hysterectomies need not worry about uterine cancer.

The question of estrogen use and breast cancer is highly controversial. Some scientists have found no risk of breast cancer associated with the use of estrogens, but a few have found a slight increase in women who have used estrogens for more than five years. For this reason we recommend that estrogens be used in as small a dose as possible under consultation by your doctor, for no more than five years, and only if it is determined that there has been sufficient bone loss to justify using it.

The only way to be sure if you have suffered bone loss to a degree that estrogen would be necessary is by new procedures that examine selected bones using a far lower dose of X-rays than previous procedures. These methods provide a rapid identification of osteoporosis, and are becoming available throughout the United States. Any woman should consider having an evaluation of her bone status performed at the time of menopause, whether or not she has symptoms. Osteoporosis frequently does not produce symptoms evident to the patient until a fall or other trauma results in a fracture, yet early treatment can be quite successful.

SUMMARY

Most Americans and people throughout the western world consume far less calcium than needed. The result is that we accelerate the epidemic of calcium-deficiency related diseases that strike in adulthood—osteoporosis, hypertension, and cancers of the intestine and breast. The risk of some very serious and disabling diseases can be reduced by increasing your level of *absorbed* calcium. Part II of *The Calcium Connection,* The Calcium Connection Program, will show you how.

4

Calcium and Blood Pressure

Fifty-eight million Americans have high blood pressure. Fourteen million Americans are presently taking medication for it. Chances are you will develop it in the future, and you might have it now. In recent years, research studies have shown a connection between blood pressure and calcium. It is yet another way in which calcium plays a crucial role in your body's health.

Blood pressure is measured by the number of millimeters a column of mercury rises in a blood pressure monitor. The first number, the systolic blood pressure, refers to the blood pressure in the arteries while the heart is contracting and racing blood into them. The second number, the diastolic blood pressure, is blood pressure between heart beats, while the heart is resting. In other words, the systolic reading measures your maximum blood pressure, and the diastolic measures your minimum blood pressure at the time the pressure is tested. A normal blood pressure reading is considered to be 120/80.

High blood pressure, though it may cause no noticeable symptoms, is very serious. It can cause kidney disease, stroke, and heart disease. Every ten points above 140/90 doubles your risk of death. This is why it is often called "the silent killer."

CALCIUM AND BLOOD PRESSURE

Several studies have shown that people who take in high amounts of calcium — 1,200 milligrams per day — have lower blood pressure and fewer health problems than people who consume smaller amounts of calcium. The typical adult woman consumes 490 milligrams of calcium per day and the typical adult man consumes 700 milligrams per day.

A government survey found that adults taking in 500 milligrams or less of calcium per day had twice the risk of hypertension as those consuming 1,500 milligrams per day or more.

The connection between calcium and blood pressure was backed by a Rancho Bernardo, California study, a fifteen-year study of adult residents of a suburban community near San Diego, initiated by Elizabeth Barrett-Connor and her colleagues at the University of California, San Diego. It showed that men who drank three or more glasses of milk a day (a food rich in calcium) had average blood pressures of 134/78, while those who consumed two glasses or less per day had average pressures of 137/81. This is a difference of three points in the systolic and diastolic blood pressure. A clinical trial of blood pressure medication by the Medical Research Council in Britain reported in the *British Medical Journal* in 1985 that a ten point drop in blood pressure cut risk of stroke virtually in half.

A test by David A. McCarron and colleagues of the Oregon Health Sciences University (1985) concluded that 1,000 milligrams of calcium taken every day for eight weeks lowered blood pressure in men and women with mild hypertension by about *five* points.

Several theories exist to explain how calcium lowers blood pressure, though none of them have yet been proven. People with normal blood pressures don't appear to lower their blood pressure by taking in higher levels of calcium. This suggests that people with hypertension suffer from a deficiency of calcium—which may mean they have trouble absorbing the calcium they take in. It may also mean that such people have abnormalities in the way their cells absorb calcium.

Vitamin D, which aids in the body's ability to absorb and use calcium, may play a role in regulation of blood pressure. A study by Mary Fran Sowers and colleagues at the University of Iowa (1985) found that women under thirty-five who took in 400 IU per day of vitamin D had systolic blood pressure six points lower than those who took in smaller amounts—an average of 111/69 compared to 117/69. They found that younger women who consumed the recommended amount of vitamin D also took in higher levels of calcium, usually from milk. Sowers attributed one point of the blood pressure drop to intake of calcium and the rest to vitamin D. Her group also analyzed the effects of body weight and alcohol intake, but found that it was vitamin D that had the greatest effect.

PREVENTING AND CONTROLLING HYPERTENSION

Large numbers of people with high blood pressure have readings only moderately above normal, between 120/80 and 150/95. If you are in this category, you may be able to reduce your blood pressure and maintain it by changing your lifestyle, instead of relying on medication. This has been confirmed by the long-term Framingham (Massachusetts) Heart Study and other studies in Illinois and Minnesota. These studies show that with goal-setting and guidance, many people who formerly took medication can maintain normal blood pressure by lifestyle changes alone. Also, people who currently need medication can often greatly reduce their dose levels if they make changes in their diet and lifestyle.

There are many ways to help lower blood pressure without drugs. First, *lose weight*. If you're 20 percent overweight, you are twice as likely to develop hypertension as someone with normal weight. Every pound you shed results in a drop of one point in blood pressure. Dieting and maintaining the lower weight is one of the most effective ways of overcoming and controlling hypertension.

Second, *reduce your use of salt*. No one with high blood pressure should eat more than 2,500 milligrams of salt a day. According to the National Academy of Sciences, most people require only 600 milligrams of salt per day.

Third, *quit smoking*. Smoking increases arteriosclerosis (hardening of the arteries) and risk of stroke.

Fourth, *raise your potassium level*. Take in 3,000 milligrams a day by including more potassium-rich foods in your diet. Appendix F lists some of the best sources of potassium. It includes a lot of foods that you probably eat anyway.

Fifth, *increase your calcium intake to the levels we recommend* (see pages 82–83). You may be able to drop your blood pressure by 8 to 10 points if you both raise your potassium intake to 3,000 milligrams and your calcium intake as recommended.

Sixth, *increase your level of vitamin D to the level we recommend* (see pages 83–84.). This amount of vitamin D may cut your blood pressure reading by several more points, particularly if you are a woman. Calcium must be absorbed in order to reduce your blood pressure and vitamin D helps your body absorb the calcium you take in and make it usable. You'll find a complete program and further guidelines to help you increase your calcium intake and absorption in the chapters to follow in *The Calcium Connection*.

MAINTAINING YOUR BLOOD PRESSURE

You may want to monitor your blood pressure to make sure it is actually being reduced by changes in your diet and lifestyle. Going to the doctor every few months to have it checked is a good idea. But blood pressure readings at the doctor's office can be misleading, as patients are often anxious in the setting of the medical office; acute anxiety temporarily raises blood pressure in some people. Although some doctors try to take the anxiety factor into account, it is difficult to judge because it varies greatly from patient to patient. If your blood pressure reads high as a result, your doctor may prescribe a course of action that is inappropriate.

The best idea for someone with high blood pressure is to buy a blood pressure measuring machine (known by the daunting name "sphygmomanometer"). They can be purchased at many pharmacies. Any doctor or nurse can teach you how to use one. You might set up an informal appointment with your physician's nurse during a quiet time at the office and take the twenty minutes or so that you'll need to learn how to use it. Then take readings in the relaxed atmosphere of your home every two weeks or so. Always take the reading at the same time of day, as blood pressure may go up or down somewhat during the day. Keep a record and you'll know how well your diet program is working. Be sure to bring your record along whenever you see your doctor; it will be valuable information for him or her about the success of your control program.

If lifestyle changes alone do not work, your doctor may prescribe medication. One common drug used is a diuretic that will cut down excessive amounts of fluid and sodium in your tissues, and increase the amount of calcium your body retains in the fluid bathing your cells. Even if you must take drugs, you can lower the dosage by increasing your calcium and potassium intake.

5

Calcium Robbers

As we've mentioned previously, there is an enormous difference between the calcium you take in daily and the amount of usable calcium that your body can absorb. Until now, all calcium tables and values printed on food packages and other calcium books have been based on crude laboratory methods. They show you how much calcium is *present*, but do not show you how much is *usable*.

Peanut butter is a perfect example of this. This popular food is listed in existing nutritional counters as having about 60 milligrams of calcium per serving. You'd think from these counters that it would therefore be a useful source of calcium. But none of the calcium in peanut butter can be absorbed and used by your body. Worse, we believe peanut butter actually *steals* 163 milligrams of calcium per serving from foods eaten with it or within a few hours of eating it.

Many foods "steal" calcium. We call such foods "calcium robbers." Calcium robbers may not wear masks or carry guns, but they can steal the calcium you take in nonetheless.

How do they do it? The molecules of calcium robbers bond extremely easily to calcium. They will readily abandon another element for calcium should they come into contact with calcium. Phytate, a molecule in certain nuts, seeds, and vegetables is a prime example. Phytate is usually bound to sodium or other elements. However, when it comes into contact with a calcium molecule, it will desert the other elements it is attached to and bond with the calcium. The problem is that when calcium is bound to phytate, the body is usually unable to unbind the two molecules, and the calcium passes through the small intestine in an unusable form until it is excreted from the body. The calcium, for all the good it has done, might just as well not have been eaten.

Similar to phytate is oxalate, another molecule that binds with calcium and makes it unusable. Many foods contain phytates and oxalates, and it is these foods that we term calcium robbers. Eating such foods with calcium-rich foods negates the potential benefits of a calcium-rich diet.

The 16 worst calcium robbers are as follows:

Robber	Mg of calcium lost per 3.5 ounce serving
Bran	−350
Swiss chard	−220
Brazil nuts	−198
Spinach	−166
Peanut butter	−163
Peanuts	−163
Shredded wheat	−157
Rhubarb	−148
Barley	−90
Tea (cup, steeped 6 minutes)	−60
Walnuts	−59
Coconut	−37
Bulgur wheat (a rough Middle Eastern cooked wheat)	−35
Beets	−34
Pecans	−19
Oats	−17

THE SPECIAL CASE OF BRAN

You may be surprised to see bran at the top of the calcium-robber list. The tendency of bran to bind calcium has long been known. Experimenters since the 1930s have fed bran-rich foods to animals to induce rickets.

Recent studies by the U.S. Department of Agriculture by Dr. June Kelsay involved feeding whole bran muffins to volunteers who were eating diets containing about 1,100 milligrams of calcium per day. One day's intake consisted of a total of one ounce of wheat bran, which was baked into muffins served two to a meal. During the experiment, the researchers found that the volunteers absorbed only 15 percent of the calcium in their diets, which was less than half of what was expected. A whopping 85 percent of the calcium was lost. As the experiment went on, the volunteers adapted to the dose of bran they received. But in the meantime, calcium absorption suffered.

Many of us eat bran-rich foods sporadically. When we do, the bran acts as a potent calcium binder and robs our bodies of at least half of the calcium we would normally absorb from other foods. A week-long binge on bran-rich food once a month could cause you to miss out on as much as 500 milligrams of the calcium you ate each day.

Because phytate was the first suspect in the test volunteers' calcium loss, scientists took out the phytate from the bran muffins used in the experiment. When the phytate was taken out of the bran, there was *still* a 20 percent decrease in calcium absorption. This is how we know that bran has a calcium-robbing effect independent of its phytate. We know that 80 percent of this calcium theft is due to phytate; the rest is due to other chemical thieves in bran, some of which have not yet been identified.

The information above may be perplexing because many doctors and nutritionists have recommended bran as a way to prevent colon cancer. But these recommendations were based mostly on comparisons of the risk of colon cancer in Africa relative to other parts of the world, including some studies which focused on fiber from fruits and vegetables, but not bran specifically. Although Africans do eat fiber-rich diets, we believe that the secret to Africa's low rates of colon cancer may be the sunlight it receives and the high levels of vitamin D that result from it—Africa is the sunniest place on the face of the earth. And we believe that bran does not especially lower the rate of colon cancer. Our review of epidemiologic results of a major, well-designed, and scrupulously conducted study reported in the *Journal of the National Cancer Institute* by Dr. Baruch Modan and his co-workers in Israel (1975) revealed that certain foods increased the risk of colon cancer. The foods seemed to fit no known pattern and the reason for their effects was not understood at the time.

The foods that were shown to increase risk of intestinal cancer in the Israeli study were:

Spinach

Walnuts

Oats

Bulgur wheat (rough Middle Eastern cooked wheat)

These are all foods we now know to be some of the worst binders of calcium in nature—and all are calcium robbers. It's no surprise that people who ate large amounts of them developed colon cancer. Some of the foods that have been most highly recommended in the past may actually be some of the worst offenders.

PROTEIN, SUGAR, AND CALCIUM

High intake of protein will also cause you to lose calcium. We need 45 to 60 grams, or about one and one half to two ounces, of protein per day to live. If you eat more than 90 grams, or three ounces, of protein per day you begin to enter a dietary range where the protein will cause calcium loss. We estimate that you will lose 50 to 70 milligrams of calcium per day for each ounce of protein you eat above three ounces. This can make a big difference if you're an avid steak or meat eater. If so, you'll need to eat additional amounts of foods in your diet that are rich in calcium to make up the difference.

Heavy intake of sugar will also cause you to lose calcium through excess excretion. The exact relationship between sugar and calcium is still being evaluated, but if you eat more than two ounces per day of sugar, honey, corn syrup, or other sugars in any form, you'll need to add calcium above the usual requirements to your diet. Until more research is completed, we recommend that you add 100 milligrams of calcium to your diet for each ounce of sugar you consume over two ounces per day. Don't forget to count the sugar in soft drinks, flavored yogurts, candy, ice cream, and syrups in canned fruit. We recommend that you eventually try to cut your intake of sugar to much less than two ounces per day.

COFFEE AND TEA

Coffee, tea, and alcohol also have an important effect on calcium absorption. One reason is that we drink so much of them. Water was once American's favorite drink, but no longer. The typical American drinks 24 ounces of coffee and soft drinks every day. Coffee is brewed in 85 percent of American homes. Many people drink ten to twenty cups per day. Step into any restaurant (often called a coffee shop) and the waitress will ask with a smile, "Coffee?" Your answer should usually be "No, thanks."

Each cup of coffee causes you to lose about 10 milligrams of calcium. This may not seem like a lot, but the loss may mean trouble if your calcium intake is already low. Most people who take in less than 500 to 600 milligrams of calcium per day are *losing* calcium from their bodies. This amount just isn't sufficient to maintain a positive calcium balance according to sophisticated studies using a tracing method based on a calcium isotope, such as that reported by Dr. H. Spencer and colleagues in the *American Journal of Medicine* (1985).

Two thirds of women in the United States and a large proportion of men don't take in as much as 600 milligrams of calcium per day. If your calcium intake is low, coffee could cause problems over time. Five cups of coffee per day could subtract 50 milligrams of calcium, calcium that will come from your bones.

If you want to keep drinking coffee, it is important that you increase your calcium intake by 10 to 20 milligrams per day for each cup of coffee that you drink.

One solution is to add nonfat or skim milk to the coffee when you drink it. Don't use cream or regular milk, however, or your fat and cholesterol intake will increase. Equally bad, or possibly even worse, is to add nondairy creamer to your coffee. You will get a large dose of coconut oil or other heavily hydrogenated oils that can cause an increase in blood cholesterol. The best answer of all is to stop drinking coffee, or cut down to a maximum of two cups per day.

There seems to be some increase of risk of certain cancers for people who drink coffee in large quantities. The effect is not dramatic, but it seems significant. We have also worked on studies of the effect of coffee on cholesterol in your blood. Perhaps surprisingly, coffee seems to increase plasma cholesterol, particularly in women. Our research group recently studied a large group of women in Southern California and found that women who drank four cups of coffee per day had plasma cholesterol levels about 15 percent higher than women who drank less than one cup per day.

There is no conclusive evidence that the harmful effects of coffee on risk of cancer or increased plasma cholesterol are due solely to caffeine, since some effects appear to be present even for decaffeinated coffee. So far it is not known which of the hundreds of chemicals found in coffee may be responsible for its health risks. But it does seem clear that the less coffee you drink, the healthier you'll be.

Many people respond to the potential health hazards of coffee with the comment, "If I can't drink coffee, I'll have tea." Americans average about four cups or glasses of iced tea or tea per month. The effect of tea on calcium in your diet depends on how the tea is prepared. If you steep the tea for a long time—six minutes—you will lose 60 milligrams of calcium for every cup you drink. Regular intake of even one cup per day could cause you to lose calcium from bone if your dietary intake of calcium is low. One solution is to steep the tea for less time. Cutting the duration of steeping to two minutes will reduce calcium loss to 20 milligrams per cup. This is still a lot and you should seriously consider cutting your intake of tea if you drink more than a cup or two per day. Herbal tea may be an answer for you, though we suggest you avoid some of the very exotic herbal teas, which may contain other toxic compounds.

What about diet or sugar-free soft drinks? Sugar-free soft drinks have become one of the most popular beverages in America. There are no data that we have found showing a large amount of calcium loss from artificially sweetened drinks.

ALCOHOL

The verdict on alcohol and its effect on calcium is not much better than that for tea or coffee. The Scotch you may look forward to each night while relaxing in your slippers with your dog has contains no calcium. People who drink a lot of alcohol tend to absorb vitamin D and calcium from their diet poorly. The result for those who drink a lot of alcohol is bone loss, even in young people. It is amazing how you can accelerate a process that leads to loss of bone by drinking alcohol, even when you are young.

Alcohol consumption has also been linked to risk of colon cancer, a relationship we observed in our study of the 1,954 Western Electric workers. Numerous other scientists have reported a similar effect. There are changes in the microscopic structure of the intestine of people who drink a lot of alcohol that make it hard for vitamin D to pass through the fine structures of the cells. The ultimate result is that the calcium is not absorbed, which causes an increase in the rate of cell division of the intestinal wall.

Moderate intake of wine may not harm calcium absorption. Recent studies show that men who drink a moderate amount of wine have no trouble absorbing calcium, although the results are not definitive. In fact, including a small amount of alcohol in your life may have positive health benefits. A number of studies have shown that people who drink a small amount of alcohol—no more than one-and-one-half glasses of wine a day, or its equivalent in beer or liquor—have 40 percent fewer deaths from heart disease and stroke than people who don't drink at all. The key is moderation. Remember that if you do consume modest amounts of alcohol, you should increase your calcium intake accordingly.

6

Calcium Transporters

Not all foods that bind calcium act as robbers. Some substances found in food act more as calcium transporters — gently carrying calcium molecules to the large intestine. Foremost of those transporters is pectin, a substance found in many fruits and vegetables, particularly in apples.

Pectin refers to both pectin and its relatives, the polysaccharides, in fruits and vegetables that aren't derived from cellulose or its relatives or starch. Pectin's relatives have cumbersome names; they are known together as water soluble noncellulose polysaccharides.

The Latin root word polysaccharide means "many sugars." These sugars are bound together so they can't be absorbed by your body. Your body is able to absorb free sugars such as fructose (fruit sugar), sucrose (table sugar), maltose (honey sugar), lactose (milk sugar), and glucose (a sugar found in carrots and other vegetables). However, the body would need a special enzyme to break the polysaccharides into smaller free sugars, and our bodies don't have the enzyme to do it. But it doesn't leave your body, either. It does something even more important.

Pectin is a faithful carrier of calcium to your large intestine. It does this with a molecular structure that looks and acts like an egg crate.

If you looked at pectin in its pure state (you can buy it at the grocery store), you'd find that it is a light-colored powder. It has a fascinating molecular structure that consists of a long chain of up to a thousand units of a simple plant acid. It looks like one of the long dragons that zigzag through a Chinese New Year parade.

If you add calcium to pectin, a gel forms. One ounce of pectin gel contains 750 *milligrams* of calcium in its molecular egg crate. Because we don't have an enzyme in our bodies that will break down pectin in our stomach or small intestine, it passes through those organs intact to the large intestine.

How does pectin in an apple work? Once the stomach has broken down the apple (which it does in about twenty minutes) the dissolved apple next moves into the small intestine, which absorbs the nutrients in the apple along its twenty-five-foot length. Most of the apple gets absorbed in a few minutes. After traveling through the small intestine, all that's left of the apple is three compounds: cellulose, lignin, and pectin. Cellulose and lignin are the compounds that make up the woody parts of the plant cell wall. They're unusable by the body and pass through untouched until they are eliminated. Pectin, however, is another matter.

Pectin next enters the large intestine, where friendly bacteria take it apart and use it as a source of fuel for themselves. They are able to do this because they have an enzyme we don't. Although bacteria eat it, it has no caloric value to us.

What, then, is the advantage of pectin? Pectin molecules embrace calcium in their egg-carton construction, making fruits and vegetables pleasantly firm and springy. The more calcium dissolved in pectin, the springier the fruit or vegetable. Scientists believe pectin's egg-crate shape is the reason it is able to safely deliver calcium to the large intestine.

Nutritionists once thought that compounds in grain, fruits, and vegetables protected the intestine by making its contents move through quickly. The theory was that shorter exposure of the foods to the intestine would cause less time for any carcinogens foods might contain to affect the cells of the intestine.

Dr. Gary Glober, a gastroenterologist, performed a study in the late 1970s of transit time, or the amount of time it takes for a meal to pass through the intestine, to find out if the theory were true. Foods can take anywhere from four to thirty-six hours to pass through the intestine of a person on a typical American diet.

Glober wanted to find out whether people who had low cancer rates of the large intestine had fast transit times. To test the idea, he compared the transit times of foods passing through the intestines of Japanese, who have a low intestinal cancer rate, with Caucasians, who have a relatively high intestinal cancer rate. Much to scientists' surprise, Glober found there was no significant difference in transit time between the low-risk cancer population and the high-risk cancer population. Research reported by Dr. D. J. A. Jenkins in the *British Medical Journal* in 1978 showed that some types of fiber actually delayed transit time.

Another theory had it that fiber increased the bulk of material in the intestine and somehow diluted the carcinogens that might be present in food. It was a plausible idea, but we now know that there are many groups of people who do not eat large amounts of grain, fruits, and vegetables and have very low rates of intestinal cancer. Japanese, for example, are a case in point. They eat a diet full of fish, polished rice, and other low-bulk foods, yet they have extremely low incidence of intestinal cancer.

After reviewing classic studies conducted by our colleagues Baruch Modan in Israel (1975); Roland Phillips, Jan Kuzma, and David Snowdon in California (1985); and Saxon Graham at Roswell Park Memorial Institute in Buffalo, New York (1978), we concluded that, unlike wheat and grains, including wheat bran, which provide little or no protection, fruits and vegetables *do* protect against intestinal cancers.

We now believe that it is pectin, the compound found in apples and other fruits and vegetables, which contributes heavily to prevention of intestinal cancer. It does so by delivering a large amount of calcium directly to the large intestine. In the acidic medium of the large intestine in many people the calcium is absorbed for use by other parts of the body, and also directly benefits the cells of the intestine's walls.

When pectin is digested by friendly acidic bacteria that live in the large intestine, it releases calcium. The calcium, in turn, appears to be slowly absorbed by the intestine while some of it reacts with fatty acids, bile salts, and other carcinogens in the intestine to form inert compounds called soaps. The soaps do not react with the lining of your large intestine, so there's no damage. Calcium binds up the attackers, rendering them unable to harm the intestinal cells. With a plentiful supply of calcium in the large intestine, the rate of cell division along the lining of the large intestine drops.

Pectins, in other words, act to transport calcium safely and effectively to the large intestine, where it can be slowly absorbed and used in the body, and where it can interact with potentially dangerous carcinogens to neutralize them.

We strongly suggest that you include in your diet as many foods that are rich in pectin as possible. Apples, oranges, lemons, limes, grapefruits, kiwis, and a wide range of fruits, as well as most vegetables, contain substantial amounts of pectin. The following is a list of some of the foods which have high amounts of pectin in them.

FOODS HIGH IN PECTIN

Food	*Milligrams per serving*
Broccoli	15
Green or white cabbage	15
Citrus fruits, with pulp	14
String beans	13
Kale	13
Brussels sprouts	13
Cucumber	13
Carrots	13
Red cabbage	11
Tomatoes	11
Cauliflower	11
Strawberries	10
Onions	8
Raspberries	8
Lima beans	8
Currants	7
Prunes	7
Apples with peel	6
Pears with peel	5
Potatoes, new	5

Source: Adapted from Hans Englyst, "Determination of Carbohydrate and Its Composition in Plant Materials," in W.P.T. James and Olof Theander (eds): *The Analysis of Dietary Fiber in Food.* New York, Marcel Dekker, Inc., 1981.

7

Your
Calcium Profile

How much calcium and vitamin D do you need in your diet to minimize the dangers of osteoporosis, high blood pressure, and cancer? As you have seen in the preceding chapters, your individual calcium and vitamin D needs will vary according to your age, whether you are a man or a woman, according to what part of the country you live in, and according to your lifestyle. The purpose of this chapter is to help design the optimal program for *you*.

Choose a quiet time and a relaxed atmosphere to fill in the profiles. You'll probably need your pocket calculator, too.

There are three profiles:

The Environmental Vitamin D Profile

The Dietary Vitamin D Profile

The Calcium Profile

The Environmental Vitamin D Profile: This profile asks a few questions about your habits and provides you with an Environmental Vitamin D score which you can use to determine how much dietary vitamin D you'll need. If you live in one of the twenty-five largest cities in the United States, you can look up your city and factor its ultraviolet light into your calculations. If you live in a smaller city you can look on a map and factor in the amount of light in your region of the country for your profile.

If, like most people, you spend a lot of time indoors, you'll need more vitamin D and calcium. If you live in an area of the country with a high level of air pollution, you'll need more, too. If you live in a northern state, you'll need more than if you live in a southern state. Filling out the profile helps to tailor the right diet for *you*. And it should only take about fifteen to twenty minutes to finish.

THE ENVIRONMENTAL VITAMIN D PROFILE

Instructions: Circle the number of points as directed for each season. You will add the points at the end of the profile to calculate your Environmental Vitamin D Score.

1. Circle the *number of points* under the best estimate of how many *minutes* you spend *outdoors** on a typical *weekday* between 9 AM and 3 PM.

	Minutes spent outdoors on a typical weekday		
Season	*Less than 8*	*8 to 15*	*More than 15*
Summer	3 points	16 points	18 points
Fall/Spring	2 points	8 points	10 points
Winter	1 point	5 points	7 points

*Outdoors in the sun or shade even on a cloudy day. Time spent in a car is not considered outdoors unless the car is a convertible with the top down.

2. Circle the *number of points* below the description which is closest to what you wear when you are outdoors between 9 AM and 3 PM on a typical *weekday*. If you spend less than 8 minutes on a typical weekday in a season, circle zero points for that season.

	What you wear when outdoors during the week		
Season	*Long sleeves, long pants or skirt*	*Short sleeves, long pants or skirt*	*Short sleeves, or no shirt, shorts*
Summer	0 points	4 points	8 points
Fall/Spring	0 points	2 points	4 points
Winter	0 points	1 point	2 points

3. Circle the *number of points* below the best estimate of how many *minutes* you spend *outdoors** on a typical *weekend* day between 9 AM and 3 PM.

Season	Minutes spent outdoors on a typical weekend day		
	Less than 8	**8 to 15**	**More than 15**
Summer	1 point	6 points	7 points
Fall/Spring	1 point	3 points	4 points
Winter	0 points	2 points	3 points

*Outdoors in the sun or shade even on a cloudy day. Time spent in a car is not considered outdoors unless the car is a convertible with the top down.

4. Circle the number of points below the description that is closest to what you wear when you are outdoors between 9 AM and 3 PM on a typical *weekend* day. If you spend less than 8 minutes on a typical weekend day in a season, circle zero points for that season.

Season	What you wear when outdoors on weekends		
	Long sleeves, long pants or skirt	Short sleeves, long pants or skirt	Short sleeves, or no shirt, shorts
Summer	0 points	2 points	3 points
Fall/Spring	0 points	1 point	2 points
Winter	0 points	0 points	1 point

Now add the numbers you have circled. Here is a worksheet.

Question	Points
1. Summer	_____
Fall/Spring	_____
Winter	_____
2. Summer	_____
Fall/Spring	_____
Winter	_____

3. Summer   _____
Fall/Spring   _____
Winter   _____

4. Summer   _____
Fall/Spring   _____
Winter   _____

Total (add column)   _____ (A)

5. Now look up the city where you live on the following list and circle your *city points* (B). If your city is not listed, choose a listed city within 30 miles. If you live elsewhere in the United States, use the map on page 71 and find the points for the area in which you live, and write the number here _____ (B).

City	City points
Baltimore MD	3
Boston MA	2
Chicago IL	2
Cleveland OH	3
Columbus OH	3
Dallas TX	5
Denver CO	3
Detroit MI	3
Honolulu HI	7
Houston TX	5
Indianapolis IN	3
Jacksonville FL	4
Los Angeles CA	3
Memphis TN	4
Milwaukee WI	2
New Orleans LA	3
New York NY	1
Philadelphia PA	2
Phoenix AZ	6

San Antonio TX	5
San Diego CA	3
San Francisco CA	2
San Jose CA	4
Seattle WA	3
Washington DC	2

Now you are ready for the last step. You may need a pocket calculator for this part.

Write your *total* points from questions 1 through 4 here ......

————— (A).

Write your *city points* (or points from map) here ————— (B).

MULTIPLY A times B and write answer here .... ————— (C).

This is your *Environmental Vitamin D Score,* and you will use it later to calculate your Total Vitamin D Score.

THE DIETARY VITAMIN D PROFILE

A portion of the vitamin D your body uses comes from diet, so a profile for it is needed. The next profile asks you how many

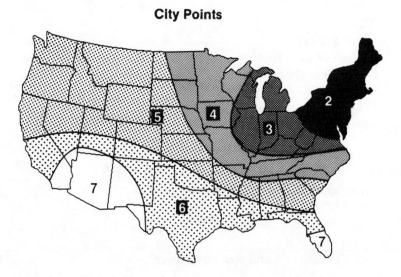

Figure 1. City points map

servings of vitamin D–containing foods you eat or drink in a typical week. Fill in the number of servings of each food that you have in a typical week. If you never have a typical week, just fill in your best estimate.

One serving of any food is 3.5 ounces. If you ate 7 ounces, you ate two servings; 11 ounces equals three servings. Less than 2 ounces equals roughly half a serving.

If you eat one serving every *two* weeks, write in ½ serving (or 0.5 if using a calculator). If you eat a food once a month, write in ¼ serving (or 0.25). Round your answer to the nearest whole number.

The Dietary Vitamin D Profile

Food	Number of servings per week	Multiply by	Points per serving	Total points
Herring	_____	×	130	= _____
Salmon	_____	×	70	= _____
Sardines, kippers or anchovies	_____	×	70	= _____
Tuna	_____	×	35	= _____
Eggs (per egg)	_____	×	7	= _____
Milk (8 oz., all types)	_____	×	15	= _____
Cheese (except cottage cheese)	_____	×	2	= _____
Margarine (2 pats)	_____	×	7	= _____
Liver (any type)	_____	×	6	= _____
Total (add column)				_____ (D)

This is your *Dietary Vitamin D Score.*

Write your *Dietary Vitamin D Score* here . . . .   _____ (D).

Write your *Environmental Vitamin D Score* here . . .   _____ (C).

ADD (D) and (C) and write total here . . . .   _____ (E).

This is your *Total Vitamin D Score.*

Interpreting your *Total Vitamin D Score.*

If your score is:	Your total vitamin D level is:	Comments:
250 or more	Desirable	You are getting enough vitamin D for a typical adult.
200 to 249	Borderline	You may need more vitamin D to be protected from the calcium deficiency diseases discussed in the book. The diets in this book will bring your intake up to the desirable level.
150 to 199	Deficient	You are not getting enough vitamin D to minimize your risk of a calcium deficiency disease. Begin diets in the book today to bring your intake up to the desirable level.
149 or less	Seriously deficient	You are getting very little vitamin D, increasing your risk of osteoporosis, and breast and intestinal cancer.

We do not recommend that you increase your exposure to the sun to raise your vitamin D level.

THE QUICK-TAKE CALCIUM PROFILE

Vitamin D can be obtained from time spent outdoors in the light, or from diet, but this isn't true for calcium. Most calcium is concentrated in a surprisingly small number of foods and beverages. Partly because of this, almost all of us consume much less calcium than we need.

By completing the following quick-take calcium profile, you will know exactly where you stand on calcium intake. The profile will take another ten minutes to complete, but it will be well worth your time.

Foods High in Calcium Write in the number of servings of each food you eat or drink in a typical week (one serving = 3.5 oz.). If you eat one serving every two weeks, write ½ (or 0.5 if using a calculator); if you eat a food once a month, write ¼ (or 0.25); less often, write zero.

High Calcium Foods
(Foods with 250 mg of calcium or more per serving)

Food	Number of servings per week
American cheese (1 oz.)	_____
Brick cheese (2 oz.)	_____
Cheddar cheese (2 oz.)	_____
Colby cheese (2 oz.)	_____
Feta cheese (2 oz.)	_____
Goat cheese (3 oz.)	_____
Gouda cheese (2 oz.)	_____
Gruyère cheese (1 oz.)	_____
Jack cheese (2 oz.)	_____
Mozzarella cheese (2 oz.)	_____
Muenster cheese (2 oz.)	_____
Parmesan cheese (1 oz.)	_____
Provolone cheese (2 oz.)	_____
Romano cheese (1 oz.)	_____
Swiss cheese (1 oz.)	_____
Buttermilk (8-oz. glass)	_____
Lowfat milk (8 oz.)	_____
Nonfat milk (8 oz.)	_____
Whole milk (8 oz.)	_____
Sardines (3 oz.)	_____
Yogurt, plain (8 oz.)	_____
Total (add column)	_____ (F)

MULTIPLY the total number of servings (F) of high calcium foods by 4 and write your answer here ....
_____ (G).

This is your number of points from *high calcium foods;* you will use this number later to calculate your total calcium intake.

Foods Moderately High in Calcium
(Foods with less than 120 mg of calcium per serving)
(One serving is 3.5 oz., except as shown.)

Food	Number of servings per week
Anchovies	_____
Artichokes	_____
Asparagus	_____
Bread and rolls	_____
Broccoli	_____
Cabbage (6 oz.)	_____
Carrots (6 oz.)	_____
Cauliflower	_____
Celery	_____
Blue or Roquefort cheese (1 oz.)	_____
Brie cheese	_____
Camembert cheese	_____
Cottage cheese	_____
Edam cheese (1 oz.)	_____
Ricotta cheese (2 oz.)	_____
Chives (1 oz.)	_____
Clams, raw	_____
Cream puff with custard	_____
Cream, half and half	_____
Cream, light whipping	_____
Cucumber	_____
Custard	_____
Eclair	_____
Egg (one)	_____
Endive	_____
Escarole	_____
Figs, dried	_____
Herring	_____
Ice cream	_____
Kale	_____
Lettuce	_____

Lobster   _____
Macaroni and cheese   _____
Muffins   _____
Mussels   _____
Oranges   _____
Oysters   _____
Pancakes   _____
Peas (6 oz.)   _____
Peapods   _____
Pears (6 oz.)   _____
Peaches (6 oz.)   _____
Pineapple (6 oz.)   _____
Pizza (1 slice)   _____
Salmon (6 oz.)   _____
Shrimp (2 oz.)   _____
Tofu   _____
Tomato   _____
Tuna   _____
Yogurt, with fruit (6 oz.)   _____

   Total (add column)   _____ (H)

   This total is your number of points from *moderately high calcium foods*.

Write *moderately high calcium food* points here ... _____ (H).

Write *high calcium food* points (from page 74) here ....
                                       _____ (G).

ADD (H) and (G) and write total here .... _____ (I).

   These are your total points from *Calcium Foods*.

Some foods bind calcium and make it unabsorbable. These are the Calcium Robbers. We have divided Calcium Robbers into two groups based on how much calcium they steal: Calcium Villains and Calcium Henchmen.

Calcium Villains
(Foods stealing 60 to 350 mg of calcium per serving)
(One serving is 3.5 oz.)

Food	Number of servings per week
Barley	_____
Bran	_____
Brazil nuts	_____
Peanut butter	_____
Peanuts	_____
Rhubarb	_____
Shredded wheat	_____
Spinach	_____
Swiss chard	_____
Tea (8 oz. steeped 6 minutes or more)	_____
Total (add column)	_____ (J)

MULTIPLY the total number of servings (J) of Calcium Villains by 2 and write your answer here . . . . _____ (K).

This is your number of points from *Calcium Villains*.

Calcium Henchmen
(Foods stealing 10 to 59 mg of calcium per serving)
(One serving is 3.5 oz.)

Food	Number of servings per week
Almonds	_____
Beets	_____
Beer (8 oz.)	_____
Coconut	_____
Coffee (8 oz.)	_____
Hard liquor (1.5 oz.)	_____
Oatmeal	_____
Pecans	_____
Tea (8 oz. steeped 5 minutes or less)	_____
Walnuts	_____
Wheat germ	_____
Total (add column)	_____ (L)

DIVIDE the total number of servings (L) of Calcium
Henchmen by 4 and write your answer here ..... _____
This total is your number of points from *Calcium Henchmen*.
Write your *Calcium Henchmen* points here .... _____ (M).
Write your *Calcium Villains* points here .... _____ (K).
ADD (M) and (K) and write the total here .... _____ (N).
        This is your total points from *Calcium Robbers*.

Calcium Score Sheet

Write total points from *Calcium Foods* here ...... _____ (I).
Write total points from *Calcium Robbers* here .... _____ (N).
SUBTRACT M from I and write answer here ..... _____ (T).
        This is your *Total Calcium Score*.

Interpreting your *Total Calcium Score*.

If your score is:	Your estimated calcium intake in milligrams per day is:	Your calcium range in milligrams is:	Your calcium intake is:
Less than 5	Less than 50	0 to 100	Seriously low
5 to 14	100	90 to 200	Seriously low
15 to 24	200	189 to 390	Seriously low
25 to 34	300	280 to 590	Seriously low
35 to 44	400	370 to 780	Seriously low
45 to 54	500	460 to 980	Seriously low
55 to 64	600	550 to 1,180	Low
65 to 74	700	640 to 1,370	Low
75 to 84	800	740 to 1,570	May be adequate
85 to 94	900	830 to 1,760	May be adequate
95 to 104	1,000	920 to 1,960	May be adequate
105 to 114	1,100	1,010 to 2,160	May be adequate
115+	1,200+	1,100 to 2,350	May be adequate

Please see chart on pages 82–83 to check your calcium need
according to your sex, age, and region.

PART II

THE

CALCIUM

CONNECTION

PROGRAM

8

The Calcium Connection Diet

Weight maintenance, even weight loss, can go hand in hand with the dietary principles we recommend. This chapter presents *two* complete diets high in both calcium and vitamin D—one for women of 2,000 calories a day, and one for men with 2,700 calories. These amounts should permit moderately active men and women to increase their calcium level to a satisfactory level, while maintaining a normal weight.

If you wish to lose weight, Chapter 9 has a 1200-calorie diet rich in calcium that will help you to lose weight. The weight-loss diet should be followed for no longer than two months at a time.

If you wish to design your own diet, you can use Tables 1 and 2. These give the daily intakes of calcium and vitamin D which we feel are needed to cut your risk of the calcium-deficiency diseases discussed in this book, including breast and colon cancer. The amounts recommended are those of the National Academy of Sciences, with additional amounts for regions with low levels of ultraviolet light, and for people at older ages.

The proper calcium and vitamin D intake for you depends on where you live and your lifestyle. The main factor you need to know to make the proper choice is your Total Vitamin D Score from your profile in Chapter 6. Look back on page 78 and see what your score is, then use the tables to select the right amount of vitamin D and calcium for you. For a quick idea of which amounts are right for you, use the diet zone map on page 71 of the Profile to determine your ultraviolet light level; then use these tables to choose your desirable vitamin D and calcium level.

The usable calcium content of most common foods is shown in the Calcium Counter of Absorbable (Usable) Calcium (Appendix A). Only a few foods contain significant amounts of vitamin D. Many ocean foods such as shark, sole, halibut, cod and shellfish which you might expect to contain vitamin D, unfortunately contain very little. The absorbable calcium content of basic foods and dishes mentioned in this book is listed Table 4, beginning on page 115.

Instructions: The tables tell you how much calcium you need each day according to where you live, your sex, age, and other factors. Just look up your city points on pages 70–71 or, if you live outside a major city, in Figure 1 on page 71. The amount of calcium you need is shown in the tables in the column under your city points.

Table 1. Desirable daily intakes of calcium (in milligrams) to prevent calcium deficiency diseases (High risk groups, ages 19 + years: Add 200 mg).*

	Your city points			
	1-2	*3*	*4-5*	*6-7*
Age				

	Your city points			
	1-2	*3*	*4-5*	*6-7*
	Men			
Age	*Desirable daily calcium intake (mg)*			
Birth to 6 months	360	360	360	360
6 months to a year	540	540	540	540
1-10 years	800	800	800	800
11-18 years	1200	1200	1200	1200
19-49 years	1000	800	800	800
50-59 years	1000	1000	800	800

Always drink 2.5 quarts of fluids a day, more when it is hot or you are perspiring. You must produce a urinary volume of 2 quarts a day. Keep dietary oxalate below 50 mg a day (see Appendix E). The information in the first table is based on the authors' research.

High risk groups include: heavy drinkers, people taking medications that reduce calcium absorption, and night workers. Do not add if you are already adding 400 mg for pregnancy or lactation. Never exceed 2000 mg intake of calcium per day unless under the advice and supervision of a doctor.

	1-2	3	4-5	6-7
60-64 years	1000	1000	1000	800
65+ years	1000	1000	1000	800

| | Women | | | |
Age	Desirable daily calcium intake (mg)			
Birth to 6 months	360	360	360	360
6 months to a year	540	540	540	540
1-10 years	800	800	800	800
11-18 years	1200	1200	1200	1200
19-49 years	1000	1000	800	800
50-59 years	1200	1000	900	800
60-64 years	1200	1200	1000	800
65+ years	1200	1200	1000	800

Pregnant or breast-feeding women, any age: Add: 400 mg per day

Table 2. Desirable daily intakes of vitamin D (in international units) to prevent calcium deficiency diseases (High risk group, ages 23 + years: Add 100 IU).†

	Your city points			
	1-2	3	4-5	6-7
	Men			
Age	Desirable daily vitamin D intake (IU)			
Birth to 18 years	400	400	400	400
19-22 years	400	350	300	300
23-64 years	200	200	200	200
64-69 years	210	200	200	200
70-79 years	220	210	200	200
80-84 years	230	220	200	200
85+ years	240	230	200	200

†*Always drink 2.5 quarts of fluids a day, more when it is hot or you are perspiring.* If you are ill or have a personal family history of kidney stones, do not modify your intake of vitamin D except on the advice of a health professional.

High risk groups include: heavy drinkers, people taking medications that reduce calcium absorption, and night workers. Do not add the 100 IU if already adding 200 IU for pregnancy or breast feeding.

Age	Women Desirable daily vitamin D intake (IU)			
Birth to 18 years	400	400	400	400
19-22 years	300	300	300	300
23-49 years	200	200	200	200
50-69 years	220	200	200	200
70-79 years	220	210	200	200
80-84 years	230	220	200	200
85+ years	240	230	200	200

Pregnant or breast-feeding women, any age: Add 200 IU

Table 3. Vitamin D Content of Selected Foods*

Food	Vitamin D (IU per 3.5 oz. serving)	Food	Vitamin D (IU per 3.5 oz. serving)
Butter	35	Milk, nonfat† (8 oz.)	100
Catfish	2,000	Milk, whole† (8 oz.)	100
Eel	4,700	Pilchard	1,500
Egg (1)	35	Salmon, Chinook	300
Flounder	40	Salmon, chum	200
Herring, canned	225	Salmon, pink	500
Herring, fresh	1,000	Salmon, red	800
Liver, beef	25	Salmon, spring	455
Liver, chicken	50	Sardines, fresh	1,500
Mackerel	500	Sardines, canned in oil	10
Margarine, fortified (2 pats)	120	Tuna	200
Milk, low-fat† (8 oz.)	100		

*The abbreviation IU stands for international units. One international unit is equivalent to 0.025 micrograms of vitamin D3.
†Almost all milk in the United States is fortified with 400 IU of vitamin D3 per quart. Most other dairy products, including half-and-half, cheese, ice cream, and yogurt are not fortified with vitamin D. Milk is generallly not fortified with vitamin D in Hawaii and in some areas. Check the label if in doubt.

THE DIETS

Each diet lasts for twenty-eight days. Both contain 60 percent complex carbohydrates, 20 percent protein, and 20 percent fat, including a large amount of omega-3 fish oils. Omega-3 fish oils have been shown to lower cholesterol in the blood and reduce risk of arteriosclerosis. A chart at the back of the diet plan lists the calcium and calories in each food in the plan.

Breakfast each day includes a La Jolla Shake, a drink that typifies the high-calcium, low-calorie, low-fat foods we recommend. Weekday lunches are simple and portable for eating away from home. Preparation of the weekday meals requires only about fifteen minutes. Weekend meals are designed for greater leisure time and may require a longer preparation time.

The cornerstone La Jolla Shake is easily prepared in the blender from milk, fruit, and tofu. Tofu, also known as soybean curd or cake, is usually associated with Oriental food. Since it is low in calories and often high in calcium—it is worthy of an important role in many recipes. You will meet it often and, we hope, pleasurably in *The Calcium Connection* diet. (At the grocery store, you will probably find tofu with the cheeses.)

To make as much of the diet's calcium available for absorption by your body, we strongly recommend you include fruits low in calcium-robbing oxalates, such as those listed below. (Appendix E gives more information about the oxalate content of different foods.)

Low Oxalate Fruits

Apples	Mangoes	Pears
Apricots	Melons	Pineapple
Bananas	Nectarines	Thompson grapes
Cherries	Oranges	
Grapefruit	Peaches	

Use fresh fruits and vegetables whenever possible. If you use frozen fruits, buy unsweetened brands. Weekday lunches can be a special problem, since many people depend on fast-food restaurants for lunch. We have found that several of the items commonly available at fast-food restaurants and office building delis fulfill our dietary recommendations, and we have included them.

A higher-calcium milk is available in grocery stores in some parts of the U.S. You may substitute it for any of the milk we list. We have suggested one glass of wine with dinner. If you don't drink alcohol, drink a glass of fruit juice or skimmed milk instead.

Drink a total of eight to ten eight-ounce glasses of fluid a day. The water you drink should contain at least 50 milligrams of calcium per quart. Some municipal water provides this. (Consult Appendix B at the back of the book for a list of the calcium content in the water of major U.S. cities). If your municipal water supply does not contain 50 milligrams of calcium per quart, Evian is one of the spring or bottled waters with high amounts of calcium you can use instead. Daily, you must also take one of the multiple vitamin and mineral supplements that provide 100 percent of the recommended daily allowance (RDA) of vitamins and minerals. You will not need a calcium supplement. Several brands fill this role; one we like is Centrum, made by Lederle Laboratories. Whichever you choose, be sure it has 100 percent of the recommended daily allowance of iron, which is 18 milligrams per day, and contains 5 milligrams of manganese.

A different menu is presented for each day—no two days are alike. An asterisk (*) next to a food means that a recipe for it is given in Part III. If no food portion or amount is listed, it means a standard 3.5-ounce portion is intended. "Milk" means nonfat milk or buttermilk, 8 ounces. We assume 8-ounce portions of juice and herb tea also. "Wine" refers to 6 ounces of table or vintage wine, not fortified wines such as sherry or port.

For vegetables, "hot" means steamed. Bread or toast assumes two slices, from loaves made from enriched white flour. Sandwiches may have enriched white, French, pita, or sourdough bread. "Oil" means olive oil, one tablespoon. "Lemon juice" also means one tablespoonful. Where other fats are called for, one teaspoon is implied. Margarine should be unsalted. Dressings assume one tablespoonful. "Rice" means white rice. "Salmon" means salmon from the Pacific Ocean.

These diets contain 800 milligrams of calcium. If your desirable intake is 1,000 to 1,200 milligrams, add high calcium foods to your diet. Another glass of nonfat milk will boost calcium intake to over 1,000 milligrams a day—while adding only 90 calories.

THE 2000 CALORIE DIET FOR WOMEN

DAY 1 / MONDAY / WEEK 1

BREAKFAST
*La Jolla Shake
Raisin toast with margarine

SNACK
Fruit
Citrus juice

LUNCH
Mixed vegetable sandwich
Fruit
Milk (6 ounces)

SNACK
Apple juice

DINNER
*Chicken Breasts Catalina
Cucumber slices with lemon
  juice
Hot rice (2 servings)
Wine
*Citrus Sorbet San Diego

SNACK
Apple juice

DAY 2 / TUESDAY / WEEK 1

BREAKFAST
*La Jolla Shake

SNACK
Fruit (2 servings)
Milk

LUNCH
Green salad with French
  dressing
Roll
Milk

SNACK
Citrus juice
Fruit

DINNER
*Vermicelli with Sauce San
  Bruno
Sliced cucumber with oil and
  vinegar
Wine
*Citrus Sorbet San Diego

SNACK
Fruit

DAY 3 / WEDNESDAY / WEEK 1

BREAKFAST
*La Jolla Shake

SNACK
Citrus juice

LUNCH
Turkey breast and tomato
    sandwich
Salad with French dressing
Milk
Fruit

DINNER
*Halibut Steak with Capers
    Capistrano
*Mushrooms and Pasta Mill
    Valley
Romaine with lemon juice
Wine
Citrus Sorbet San Diego

SNACK
Fruit

DAY 4 / THURSDAY / WEEK 1

BREAKFAST
*La Jolla Shake

SNACK
Bagel with margarine
Citrus juice

LUNCH
Salad
Salmon salad sandwich

DINNER
*Fettucine Sausalito
Sliced mushrooms and
    cucumber with oil, lemon
    juice, and herbs
Roll
Wine
*Citrus Sorbet San Diego

DAY 5 / FRIDAY / WEEK 1

BREAKFAST
*La Jolla Shake
Toast with margarine,
  cinnamon, and fructose

SNACK
Citrus juice

LUNCH
Egg salad sandwich
Milk (4 ounces)
Fruit (2 servings)

DINNER
*Caesar Salad Coronado
Roll with margarine
Wine
*Pears Pearldale

SNACK
Fruit
*Poppyseed Dressing
  California

DAY 6 / SATURDAY / WEEK 1

BREAKFAST
*La Jolla Shake
Toast with margarine and
  jam

LUNCH
Fruit salad
*Poppyseed Dressing
  California
Rolls (2)
Citrus juice

SNACK
Apple juice

DINNER
*Seafood Strata Sunset Beach
Romaine, tomato, and
  cucumber with oil
  (1 teaspoon), vinegar, and
  herbs
Wine
*Fresh Fruit Sorbet Stovepipe
  Wells (1½ servings)

SNACK
Fruit

DAY 7 / SUNDAY / WEEK 1

BREAKFAST
*La Jolla Shake

SNACK
Apple juice

LUNCH
*Chef's Salad Carnelian Bay
Milk (6 ounces)
*Apple Crumble Julian

SNACK
Citrus juice

DINNER
*Pizza Palomar
Sliced cucumber with oil and
  vinegar
Wine
*Citrus Sorbet San Diego
  (2 servings)

DAY 8 / MONDAY / WEEK 2

BREAKFAST
*La Jolla Shake
English muffin with jam and
  margarine

SNACK
Citrus juice

LUNCH
Mixed vegetable sandwich
Milk (4 ounces)
Fruit
*Poppyseed Dressing
  California

DINNER
*Vegetable Loaves Venice
Corn with margarine
  (2 servings)
Butterhead lettuce, tomatoes,
  and mushrooms with oil
  (1 teaspoon), vinegar, and
  herbs
Wine
*Citrus Sorbet San Diego

SNACK
Fruit

DAY 9 / TUESDAY / WEEK 2

BREAKFAST
*La Jolla Shake
Bagel with margarine

SNACK
Fruit
Citrus juice

LUNCH
Green salad with French
    dressing
Chicken salad sandwich
Fruit (2 servings)

DINNER
*Salmon Shell Beach
Hot baby new potatoes and
    peas tossed with oil,
    vinegar, and herbs
Wine
Fruit

SNACK
Apple juice

DAY 10 / WEDNESDAY / WEEK 2

BREAKFAST
*La Jolla Shake
English muffin with
    margarine and jam

SNACK
Fruit

LUNCH
Mixed vegetable sandwich
Fruit

DINNER
*Spaghetti Santa Nella
Cucumber with oil
    (2 tablespoons), lemon
    juice, and herbs
Wine
*Citrus Sorbet San Diego

SNACK
Fruit

DAY 11 / THURSDAY / WEEK 2

BREAKFAST
*La Jolla Shake
Roll

SNACK
Milk
Roll

LUNCH
Green salad with French
    dressing
Tuna salad sandwich

DINNER
Chicken breasts grilled with
    oil, lemon juice, ginger,
    and rosemary (2 servings)
Pasta (2 servings) with
    margarine
Tomato and cucumber with
    oil and lemon juice
Wine
*Citrus Sorbet San Diego
    (2 servings)

SNACK
Fruit

DAY 12 / FRIDAY / WEEK 2

BREAKFAST
*La Jolla Shake

SNACK
Fruit (2 servings)
Milk (6 ounces)

LUNCH
Chicken salad sandwich
Fruit
Citrus fruit

SNACK
Apple juice

DINNER
*Sea Salad Seal Beach
Pasta with margarine
    (2 servings)
Wine

SNACK
Fruit

DAY 13 / SATURDAY / WEEK 2

BREAKFAST
*La Jolla Shake

SNACK
Fruit

LUNCH
Turkey breast and tomato
  sandwich
Milk (4 ounces)
Citrus juice
Fruit (2 servings)

DINNER
*Linguine Casa Loma
Wine
*Citrus Sorbet San Diego

SNACK
Fruit

DAY 14 / SUNDAY / WEEK 2

BREAKFAST
*La Jolla Shake

SNACK
Fruit
Roll with margarine

LUNCH
*Vegetable Caviar Viola
Bread
Fruit
Milk (4 ounces)

SNACK
Citrus juice

DINNER
*Pasta Fiesta Island
Rolls (2) with margarine
Wine
Fruit
*Fresh Fruit Sorbet Stovepipe
  Wells

DAY 15 / MONDAY / WEEK 3

BREAKFAST
*La Jolla Shake

SNACK
Fruit
Citrus juice

LUNCH
Fruit salad (2 servings)
Roll
Milk

SNACK
Apple juice

DINNER
*Spaghettini and Clam Sauce
    Pismo Beach
Sliced cucumber and
    tomatoes with oil and
    lemon juice
Wine
*Citrus Sorbet San Diego

DAY 16 / TUESDAY / WEEK 3

BREAKFAST
*La Jolla Shake

SNACK
Fruit
Citrus juice

LUNCH
Pasta salad (2 servings)
Fruit
Milk

SNACK
Apple juice

DINNER
*Chicken Kabobs Malibu
    Colony
Hot corn on the cob
    (2 servings) with
    margarine
Lettuce with French dressing
Wine
*Baked Apples Applegate

SNACK
Fruit

DAY 17 / WEDNESDAY / WEEK 3

BREAKFAST
*La Jolla Shake

SNACK
Fruit roll
Citrus juice

LUNCH
Chicken salad sandwich
Milk

DINNER
*Trout Twin Bridges
Hot baby turnips, pasta, and
    carrots with oil, lemon
    juice, and herbs
Wine
*Citrus Sorbet San Diego

DAY 18 / THURSDAY / WEEK 3

BREAKFAST
*La Jolla Shake

SNACK
Milk (4 ounces)

LUNCH
Tuna salad sandwich
Green salad with garlic
    dressing
Citrus juice

DINNER
*Pasta Nuevo
Cherry tomatoes and
    mushroom slices with
    lemon juice and herbs
Wine
*Citrus Sorbet San Diego

SNACK
Apple juice

DAY 19 / FRIDAY / WEEK 3

BREAKFAST
*La Jolla Shake

SNACK
Fruit
Fruit muffin
Milk

LUNCH
Turkey breast and tomato
    sandwich
Citrus juice
Fruit

SNACK
Apple juice

DINNER
*Sole Marina del Rey
    (2 servings)
*Rice Pilaf Ranchita
    (2 servings)
Cucumber slices with oil and
    lemon juice
Wine
*Citrus Sorbet San Diego

DAY 20 / SATURDAY / WEEK 3

BREAKFAST
*La Jolla Shake
Fruit muffin

LUNCH
Pasta salad
Apple juice

SNACK
*Citrus Sorbet San Diego
    (2 servings)

DINNER
*Cream of Champagne Soup
    Cardiff (half serving)
Hot whole artichoke
*Mayonnaise Malibu
Steamed lobster tails
    (2 servings)
Drawn butter (2 tablespoons)
French roll
Champagne
Kiwi and papaya
*Fruit Salad Dressing Soledad
    (2 tablespoons)

DAY 21 / SUNDAY / WEEK 3

BREAKFAST
*La Jolla Shake
Raisin bread (1 slice)

LUNCH
*Eggs Exeter
*Blueberry Bun Bass Lake
Milk (6 ounces)
*Poppyseed Dressing
  California with fruit

DINNER
Salmon grilled with oil
  (1 teaspoon), lemon juice,
  and cilantro leaves
Romaine and tomato salad
  with lemon juice
Corn muffin
Wine
*Citrus Sorbet San Diego
  (2 servings)

SNACK
Fruit

DAY 22 / MONDAY / WEEK 4

BREAKFAST
*La Jolla Shake

SNACK
Fruit
  (2 servings)
Citrus juice

LUNCH
Fruit salad
Corn muffins (2)
Milk (6 ounces)

SNACK
Apple juice

DINNER
Broiled chicken breast
  (2 servings)
Hot baby potatoes and baby
  peas, tossed with margarine
  (2 teaspoons) and herbs
Wine
*Peaches Pacifica

SNACK
Apple juice

DAY 23 / TUESDAY / WEEK 4

BREAKFAST
*La Jolla Shake

SNACK
Fruit muffin
Fruit

LUNCH
Mixed vegetable sandwich
Fruit
Milk

DINNER
*Egg Salad El Granada
Garlic bread with margarine
   (1 slice)
Wine
Fruit
*Poppyseed Dressing
   California

SNACK
*Citrus Sorbet San Diego
   (2 servings)

DAY 24 / WEDNESDAY / WEEK 4

BREAKFAST
*La Jolla Shake

SNACK
Fruit
Citrus juice

LUNCH
Pasta salad (2 servings)
Roll
Milk
Fruit

SNACK
Apple juice

DINNER
*Codfish Blue Lake
   (2 servings)
*Red Cabbage Reseda
Hot new potatoes
Wine
*Citrus Sorbet San Diego

SNACK
Fruit

DAY 25 / THURSDAY / WEEK 4

BREAKFAST
*La Jolla Shake

SNACK
Fruit

LUNCH
Salmon salad sandwich
Milk (4 ounces)
Fruit (2 servings)

DINNER
*Linguine and Cauliflower
   Californio
Wine
*Citrus Sorbet San Diego
   (2 servings)

SNACK
Apple juice

DAY 26 / FRIDAY / WEEK 4

BREAKFAST
*La Jolla Shake

SNACK
Fruit
Citrus juice

LUNCH
Turkey breast and tomato
   sandwich
Milk (4 ounces)
Fruit (2 servings)

SNACK
Apple juice

DINNER
*Vegetables Chinatown
Wine
*Citrus Sorbet San Diego

SNACK
Fruit
*Poppyseed Dressing
   California

DAY 27 / SATURDAY / WEEK 4

BREAKFAST
*La Jolla Shake
Fruit roll

SNACK
Fruit

LUNCH
Chicken salad sandwich
Milk (4 ounces)
Fruit
*Poppyseed Dressing
   California

SNACK
Apple juice

DINNER
*Oyster Sandwich Orleans
Tomato slices
Wine
*Citrus Sorbet San Diego

SNACK
Apple juice

DAY 28 / SUNDAY / WEEK 4

BREAKFAST
*La Jolla Shake

SNACK
Fruit

LUNCH
*Stuffed Eggs Escondido
Pasta salad
Milk (4 ounces)

DINNER
*Tacos Truckee
*Gazpacho Gonzales
   (1½ servings)
Wine
*Citrus Sorbet San Diego
   (2 servings)

SNACK
Apple juice

THE 2700 CALORIE DIET FOR MEN

DAY 1 / MONDAY / WEEK 1

BREAKFAST
*La Jolla Shake
Raisin toast with margarine
  and jam
Fruit

SNACK
Citrus juice

LUNCH
Mixed vegetable sandwich
  with mayonnaise
Fruit
Milk

SNACK
Apple juice

DINNER
*Chicken Breasts Catalina
Hot rice (2 servings)
Cucumber slices with oil,
  lemon juice, and herbs
Wine
*Citrus Sorbet San Diego
  (2 servings)

SNACK
Fruit
Apple juice

DAY 2 / TUESDAY / WEEK 1

BREAKFAST
*La Jolla Shake
Fruit

SNACK
Fruit
Milk

LUNCH
Green salad with French
  dressing (3 servings)
Roll
Citrus juice

SNACK
Fruit

DINNER
*Vermicelli with Sauce San
  Bruno
Sliced cucumber with oil
  (1 tablespoon), vinegar, and
  herbs
Wine
*Citrus Sorbet San Diego
  (2 servings)

SNACK
Fruit

DAY 3 / WEDNESDAY / WEEK 1

BREAKFAST
*La Jolla Shake
Toast and jam

SNACK
Citrus juice

LUNCH
Egg salad sandwich
Salad with French dressing
Milk (4 ounces)
Fruit

DINNER
*Halibut Steak with Capers
  Capistrano
*Mushrooms and Pasta Mill
  Valley
Romaine with lemon juice
  and olive oil (1 tablespoon)
Wine
*Citrus Sorbet San Diego
  (2 servings)

SNACK
Fruit

DAY 4 / THURSDAY / WEEK 1

BREAKFAST
*La Jolla Shake
Bagel with margarine

SNACK
Citrus juice

LUNCH
Salmon salad sandwich
Milk (4 ounces)
Fruit

SNACK
Apple juice

DINNER
*Fettucine Sausalito
Mushroom and cucumber
  slices with oil
  (2 tablespoons), lemon
  juice, and herbs
Roll
Wine
*Citrus Sorbet San Diego
  (2 servings)

DAY 5 / FRIDAY / WEEK 1

BREAKFAST
*La Jolla Shake
Toast, with margarine,
  fructose, and cinnamon

SNACK
Citrus juice

LUNCH
Turkey breast and tomato
  sandwich
Fruit (2 servings)

SNACK
Apple Juice

DINNER
*Caesar Salad Coronado
Rolls with margarine (2)
Wine
*Pears Pearldale (2 servings)

SNACK
Fruit (2 servings)
*Poppyseed Dressing
  California (2 tablespoons)
*Citrus Sorbet San Diego

DAY 6 / SATURDAY / WEEK 1

BREAKFAST
*La Jolla Shake
Toast with margarine and
  jam

LUNCH
Fruit salad
*Poppyseed Dressing
  California
Fruit rolls (2)
Citrus juice

SNACK
Apple juice

DINNER
*Seafood Strata Sunset Beach
Romaine, tomato, and
  cucumber with oil
  (2 tablespoons), vinegar,
  and herbs
Wine
*Citrus Sorbet San Diego
  (2 servings)

SNACK
Fruit

DAY 7 / SUNDAY / WEEK 1

BREAKFAST
*La Jolla Shake

SNACK
Apple juice

LUNCH
*Chef's Salad Carnelian Bay
Milk (4 ounces)
*Apple Crumble Julian
  (2 servings)

SNACK
Citrus juice

DINNER
*Pizza Palomar
Sliced cucumber with oil,
  vinegar, and herbs
Wine
*Citrus Sorbet San Diego
  (2 servings)

DAY 8 / MONDAY / WEEK 2

BREAKFAST
*La Jolla Shake
English muffin with jam and
  margarine

SNACK
Citrus juice

LUNCH
Mixed vegetable sandwich
  with dressing
Fruit (2 servings)
*Poppyseed Dressing
  California (2 tablespoons)

SNACK
Fruit

DINNER
*Vegetable Loaves Venice
Corn with margarine
  (2 servings)
Lettuce, tomato wedges, and
  sliced mushrooms with oil
  (2 tablespoons), vinegar,
  and herbs
Wine
*Citrus Sorbet San Diego
  (2 servings)

SNACK
Apple juice

DAY 9 / TUESDAY / WEEK 2

BREAKFAST
*La Jolla Shake
Bagel with margarine and
  jam (2 tablespoons)
Fruit

SNACK
Citrus juice
Cinnamon roll

LUNCH
Green salad with French
  dressing (2 servings)
Chicken salad sandwich
Fruit (2 servings)

DINNER
*Salmon Shell Beach
Hot baby new potatoes and
  baby peas tossed with oil,
  vinegar, and herbs
Wine
*Peaches Pacifica

SNACK
*Citrus Sorbet San Diego
  (2 servings)

DAY 10 / WEDNESDAY / WEEK 2

BREAKFAST
*La Jolla Shake
English muffin with
  margarine and jam

SNACK
Fruit (2 servings)

LUNCH
Mixed vegetable sandwich (2)
Fruit
Apple juice

DINNER
*Spaghetti Santa Nella
Cucumber with oil
  (2 tablespoons), lemon
  juice, and herbs
Wine
*Citrus Sorbet San Diego
  (2 servings)

DAY 11 / THURSDAY / WEEK 2

BREAKFAST
*La Jolla Shake
Roll

SNACK
Roll
Citrus juice

LUNCH
Green salad with French
  dressing (2 servings)
Tuna salad sandwich
Milk

DINNER
Chicken breasts grilled with
  oil, lemon juice, ginger,
  and rosemary
Pasta (2 servings)
Tomato and cucumber with
  oil (2 tablespoons), vinegar,
  and herbs
Wine
*Citrus Sorbet San Diego
  (2 servings)

SNACK
Fruit

DAY 12 / FRIDAY / WEEK 2

BREAKFAST
*La Jolla Shake
Fruit (2 servings)

SNACK
Milk (4 ounces)
Fruit

LUNCH
Chicken salad sandwich with
  dressing
Fruit
Citrus juice

SNACK
Apple juice
Fruit roll

DINNER
*Sea Salad Seal Beach, in
  tomato shells (1½ servings)
Pasta with margarine
  (2 servings)
Wine
*Citrus Sorbet San Diego
  (2 servings)

SNACK
Apple juice

DAY 13 / SATURDAY / WEEK 2

BREAKFAST
*La Jolla Shake
Fruit

SNACK
Apple juice

LUNCH
Turkey breast and tomato
  sandwich (2)
Fruit (2 servings)

SNACK
Citrus juice

DINNER
*Linguine Casa Loma
Wine
*Citrus Sorbet San Diego
  (2 servings)

DAY 14 / SUNDAY / WEEK 2

BREAKFAST
*La Jolla Shake
Fruit
Roll with margarine

LUNCH
*Vegetable Caviar Viola
Bread
Fruit
Milk (4 ounces)

SNACK
Citrus juice

DINNER
*Pasta Fiesta Island
Rolls with margarine (2)
Wine
*Citrus Sorbet San Diego
  (2 servings)

SNACK
Apple juice

DAY 15 / MONDAY / WEEK 3

BREAKFAST
*La Jolla Shake
Fruit

SNACK
Citrus juice

LUNCH
Fruit salad with apple
  (2 servings)
Roll
Milk

SNACK
Apple juice

DINNER
*Spaghettini with Clam Sauce
  Pismo Beach
Butterhead lettuce,
  cucumber, and tomato with
  oil (2 tablespoons), lemon
  juice, and herbs
Milk
*Citrus Sorbet San Diego
  (2 servings)

SNACK
Apple juice

DAY 16 / TUESDAY / WEEK 3

BREAKFAST
*La Jolla Shake
Fruit

SNACK
Citrus juice

LUNCH
Pasta salad (2 servings)
Fruit
Milk (6 ounces)

SNACK
Apple juice

DINNER
*Chicken Kabobs Malibu
  Colony
Hot corn on the cob with
  margarine (2 servings)
Green salad with French
  dressing
Wine
*Baked Apples Applegate
  (2 servings)

SNACK
*Citrus Sorbet San Diego
  (2 servings)

DAY 17 / WEDNESDAY / WEEK 3

BREAKFAST
*La Jolla Shake
Fruit

SNACK
Fruit roll with jam
Citrus juice

LUNCH
Chicken salad sandwich
Fruit
Milk (6 ounces)

SNACK
Apple juice

DINNER
*Trout Twin Bridges
Hot baby turnips, baby
    carrots, and cooked pasta
    with oil (2 tablespoons),
    lemon juice, and herbs
Wine
*Citrus Sorbet San Diego
    (2 servings)

SNACK
Fruit

DAY 18 / THURSDAY / WEEK 3

BREAKFAST
*La Jolla Shake
Fruit

SNACK
Cinnamon roll

LUNCH
Tuna salad sandwich
Green salad with garlic
    dressing
Fruit
Citrus juice

DINNER
*Pasta Nuevo (1½ servings)
Sliced tomato and
    mushrooms with lemon
    juice, oil (1 tablespoon),
    and herbs
Wine
*Citrus Sorbet San Diego
    (2 servings)

SNACK
Apple juice

DAY 19 / FRIDAY / WEEK 3

BREAKFAST
*La Jolla Shake
Fruit

SNACK
Fruit muffin with jam
Milk

LUNCH
Turkey breast and tomato
  sandwich with dressing
Citrus juice
Fruit

SNACK
Apple juice

DINNER
*Sole Marina del Rey
  (2 servings)
*Rice Pilaf Ranchita
  (2 servings)
Cucumber slices with oil
  (1 tablespoon), lemon juice,
  and herbs
Wine
*Citrus Sorbet San Diego
  (2 servings)

SNACK
Apple juice

DAY 20 / SATURDAY / WEEK 3

BREAKFAST
*La Jolla Shake
Fruit muffins (2) with jam

LUNCH
Pasta salad (2 servings)
Apple juice
*Citrus Sorbet San Diego

DINNER
*Cream of Champagne Soup
  Cardiff (half serving)
Hot whole artichoke

*Mayonnaise Malibu
Steamed lobster tails
  (2 servings)
Drawn butter (2 tablespoons)
French roll
Champagne
Kiwi and papaya
*Fruit Salad Dressing Soledad
  (2 tablespoons)

SNACK
Apple juice

DAY 21 / SUNDAY / WEEK 3

BREAKFAST
*La Jolla Shake
Raisin toast and jam
Fruit

SNACK
Apple juice

LUNCH
*Eggs Exeter
*Blueberry Bun Bass Lake
Fruit
*Poppyseed Dressing
California (2 tablespoons)
Citrus juice

SNACK
Apple juice

DINNER
Salmon grilled with oil
(1 tablespoon), lemon juice,
and cilantro leaves
Romaine and tomato with oil
(2 tablespoons), lemon
juice, and herbs
Roll
Wine
*Citrus Sorbet San Diego
(2 servings)

SNACK
Fruit

DAY 22 / MONDAY / WEEK 4

BREAKFAST
*La Jolla Shake
Fruit (2 servings)

SNACK
Citrus juice

LUNCH
Fruit salad (2 servings)
Rolls (2)
Milk (6 ounces)

SNACK
Apple juice

DINNER
Broiled chicken breast
(2 servings)
Hot baby new potatoes and
baby peas, tossed with
margarine (2 teaspoons)
and herbs
Wine
*Peaches Pacifica (2 servings)

SNACK
*Citrus Sorbet San Diego
(2 servings)

DAY 23 / TUESDAY / WEEK 4

BREAKFAST
*La Jolla Shake
Fruit

SNACK
Fruit muffin
Citrus juice

LUNCH
Mixed vegetable sandwich (2)
  with dressing
Fruit
Milk (4 ounces)

DINNER
*Egg Salad El Granada
Garlic bread with margarine
  (2 servings)
Wine
Fruit
*Poppyseed Dressing
  California

SNACK
*Citrus Sorbet San Diego
  (2 servings)

DAY 24 / WEDNESDAY / WEEK 4

BREAKFAST
*La Jolla Shake
Fruit

SNACK
Citrus juice

LUNCH
Pasta salad (2 servings)
Roll with jam
Green salad with garlic
  dressing (2 tablespoons)
Milk
Fruit

SNACK
Apple juice

DINNER
*Codfish Blue Lake
  (2 servings)
*Red Cabbage Reseda
Hot new potatoes
Wine
*Citrus Sorbet San Diego
  (2 servings)

SNACK
Fruit

DAY 25 / THURSDAY / WEEK 4

BREAKFAST
*La Jolla Shake
Fruit

SNACK
Fruit (2 servings)

LUNCH
Salmon salad sandwich
Mixed salad with French
  dressing (2 servings)
Milk (4 ounces)
Fruit (2 servings)

SNACK
Apple juice

DINNER
*Linguine and Cauliflower
  Californio
Wine
*Citrus Sorbet San Diego
  (2 servings)

SNACK
Apple juice

DAY 26 / FRIDAY / WEEK 4

BREAKFAST
*La Jolla Shake
Fruit

SNACK
Citrus juice

LUNCH
Turkey breast and tomato
  sandwich with dressing
Milk
Fruit (2 servings)

SNACK
Apple juice

DINNER
*Vegetables Chinatown
Wine
Fruit
*Poppyseed Dressing
  California

SNACK
*Citrus Sorbet San Diego
  (2 servings)
Apple juice

DAY 27 / SATURDAY / WEEK 4

BREAKFAST
*La Jolla Shake
Fruit roll

SNACK
Fruit

LUNCH
Chicken Salad Sandwich
  with dressing
Fruit (2 servings)
*Poppyseed Dressing
  California (2 servings)
Milk (4 ounces)

SNACK
Apple juice

DINNER
*Oyster Sandwich Orleans
Tomato slices with oil
  (1 tablespoon) and vinegar
Wine
*Citrus Sorbet San Diego
  (2 servings)

SNACK
Apple juice

DAY 28 / SUNDAY / WEEK 4

BREAKFAST
*La Jolla Shake
Fruit

SNACK
Apple juice

LUNCH
*Stuffed Eggs Escondido
Pasta salad (3 servings)
Lettuce with oil
  (1 tablespoon) and lemon
  juice
Milk (4 ounces)

DINNER
*Tacos Truckee
*Gazpacho Gonzales
  (2 servings)
Green salad with oil
  (1 tablespoon) and vinegar
Wine
*Citrus Sorbet San Diego
  (2 servings)

SNACK
Apple juice

Table 4 shows the calcium-to-calorie rations of basic foods and
dishes mentioned in the diets in this chapter and Chapter 5.

TABLE 4. CALCIUM/CALORIE RATIO

(One serving is generally considered 3.5 ounces, though serving sizes may vary according to the recipe.)

Food/Recipe per serving	Calcium (mg)	Calories	Calcium / Calorie ratio	Diets with ° recipes	
				2000/ 2700 cal	1200 cal
Yogurt (3.5 oz)	190	50	3.8		
Kale (3.5 oz)	178	53	3.4		
Nonfat milk (8-oz. glass)	271	81	3.3		
Broccoli (3.5 oz)	103	32	3.2		
Parmesan cheese (3.5 oz)	1140	393	2.9		
*Anchovy Spread Angel's Camp	196	75	2.6	✓	
Grapefruit (3.5 oz)	41	16	2.6		
Swiss cheese (3.5 oz)	925	370	2.5		
Butterhead lettuce (3.5 oz)	35	14	2.5		
*Anchovy Spread Avalon	273	118	2.3		
Sardines, canned with tomato sauce (3.5 oz)	449	197	2.3		
*Vegetable-Yogurt Loaf Tahoe	504	220	2.3		
*Cream of Champagne Soup Cardiff	531	241	2.2	✓	✓
Cabbage (3.5 oz)	49	24	2.0		
Artichoke (3.5 oz)	51	25	2.0		
*Vegetable-Yogurt Loaf Tecopa	186	97	1.9	✓	
Cheddar cheese (3.5 oz)	750	398	1.9		

Tofu (3.5 oz)	128	72	1.8		
*Vegetable Caviar Ventura	300	172	1.7		
*La Jolla Shake	228	136	1.7	✓	✓
Cucumber (3.5 oz)	25	15	1.7		
*Cauliflower with Crab Carmel	98	62	1.6		
*Broccoli Tierrasanta	233	142	1.6		✓
*Seafood Strata Santa Monica	940	609	1.5		
*Salmon Mold San Carlos	367	241	1.5		✓
*Baked Broccoli Bel Air	175	116	1.5		✓
*Salmon Shell Beach	310	208	1.5	✓	✓
Eastern oysters (3.5 oz)	94	66	1.4		
*Omelet Ojai	293	210	1.4		
*Salmon Santa Cruz	634	448	1.4		
*Pasta Madera	519	365	1.4		
*Tacos Temecula	655	465	1.4		
*Cheese Log Canoga	404	287	1.4		✓
*Salmon Seacliff	448	335	1.3		✓
*Mayonnaise Malibu	49	37	1.3	✓	✓
*Caesar Salad Salinas	401	316	1.3		
*Vegetable Loaves Venice	201	166	1.2	✓	
*Albacore Parmesan Alhambra	328	274	1.2		
*Broccoli Berkeley	229	194	1.2		
*Gourmet Cheese Dressing Gringo (1T)	53	47	1.1		✓

*Chef's Salad Loma Linda	457	412	1.1	
*Vegetable Caviar Viola	97	90	1.1	✓ ✓
Salmon, Pacific	180	170	1.1	
*Cheese Dip Del Mar	123	129	1.0	
*Zucchini-Mushroom Salad San Joaquin	86	84	1.0	
*Pasta Shells Siciliano	487	498	1.0	✓
*Seafood Strata Sunset Beach	356	373	1.0	✓
*Salmon Sausalito	227	238	1.0	✓
*Lasagna Little Italy	779	825	0.9	✓
Ricotta cheese (3.5 oz)	160	170	0.9	
*Stuffed Eggs Escondido	128	139	0.9	✓ ✓
*Chicken Cheddar Casserole Chico	406	444	0.9	
*Red Cabbage Reseda	66	73	0.9	✓ ✓
*Cauliflower (3.5 oz)	24	27	0.9	
Cottage cheese (3.5 oz)	94	106	0.9	
*Red Snapper with Vegetables Vista	172	194	0.9	
*Oysters Oceanside	221	249	0.9	
*Eggs Elsinore	178	193	0.9	
*Lasagna Chiampino	652	800	0.8	
*Pasta Pensaquitos	294	352	0.8	✓
Orange (3.5 oz)	40	49	0.8	
*Fruit Parfait Pala	139	172	0.8	
*Ravioli Riverside	391	487	0.8	✓
*Chef's Salad Half Moon Bay	265	337	0.8	✓
*Chicken Breasts Santa Ysabel	119	158	0.8	✓

*Pasta Garden Vegetable San Fernando	144	220	0.7		
*Tacos Truckee	203	287	0.7	✓	
Shrimp (3.5 oz)	63	91	0.7		
*Linguine Lafayette	268	392	0.7		✓
*Broccoli Soup Balboa	154	221	0.7		
*Omelet Ocotillo	127	188	0.7	✓	
*Scallops San Simeon	94	141	0.7	✓	
*Pasta Broccoli Bolinas	273	488	0.6		
*Shrimp in Tomato Beds Tehama	214	313	0.7		
*Shrimp Laguna Beach	139	217	0.6		✓
*Sea Salad Seal Beach	106	170	0.6	✓	✓
*Oysters Pirate's Cove	138	222	0.6		✓
*Caesar Salad Coronado	139	226	0.6	✓	✓
*Chicken Kabobs Malibu Colony	148	242	0.6	✓	✓
*Chicken Parmesan Petaluma	168	259	0.6		
Tomato (3.5 oz)	13	22	0.6		
*Lasagna Live Oak	406	702	0.6		✓
*Fettucine Sunland	161	315	0.7		✓
*Fruit Salad Dressing Soledad (1 tablespoon)	17	31	0.5	✓	✓
*Whipped Delight Whittier	63	115	0.5		
*Spaghetti San Francisco	174	325	0.5		✓
*Pasta and Cheese Cucamonga	407	789	0.5		

*Chef's Salad Carnelian Bay	144	294	0.5	✓	
*Chicken Carlsbad	123	252	0.5		✓
*Turnips Tiburon	134	277	0.5		
*Oyster Sandwich Orleans	171	354	0.5	✓	
*Croquettes Campo	141	295	0.5		
*Compote Apple Valley	56	119	0.5		✓
*Chickpeas Calico	213	458	0.5		
Crab (3.5 oz)	43	93	0.5		
*Shrimp Dip Diamond Springs	78	169	0.5		✓
*Shad Shelter Cove	169	368	0.5		
*Sauce Rancho Mirage	187	445	0.4		
*Linguine Casa Loma	283	689	0.4	✓	
*Pizza Palomar	211	516	0.4	✓	
Plums, Damson (3.5 oz)	26	66	0.4		
*Fettucini Felicita Park	247	681	0.4		
*Spaghetti Santa Nella	206	569	0.4	✓	
*Chicken Breasts Catalina	48	134	0.4	✓	
*Spaghettini with Clam Sauce Catalina	223	629	0.4		
*Eggs Exeter	41	116	0.4	✓	✓
*Shrimp Barbecue Monterey	173	495	0.3		
*Vermicelli with Sauce Sorrento Valley	217	650	0.3		
Egg (3.5 oz)	54	163	0.3		
Scallops (3.5 oz)	26	81	0.3		
Lobster (3.5 oz)	29	91	0.3		
*Gazpacho Gonzales	34	110	0.3	✓	

*Vegetables Chinatown	186	633	0.3	✓	
*Cherries Chula Vista	108	344	0.3		✓
*Linguine and Cauliflower Californio	155	562	0.3	✓	
Watermelon (3.5 oz)	7	26	0.3		
*Poppyseed Dressing California	11	41	0.3	✓	✓
*Trout Twin Bridges	72	275	0.3	✓	
*Shrimp with Pasta San Luis Rey	96	391	0.2		✓
Blueberries (3.5 oz)	15	62	0.2		
Peach (3.5 oz)	9	38	0.2		
*Oyster Cod Ocean Beach	95	474	0.2		
*Fruit Sorbet Rancho Santa Fe	24	122	0.2		✓
*Blackberry Pudding Bay Bridge	58	301	0.2		
*Pasta Nuevo	94	493	0.2	✓	
Rainbow trout (3.5 oz)	36	195	0.2		
*Blueberry Buns Bass Lake	45	271	0.2	✓	
*Egg Salad El Granada	62	375	0.2	✓	
Thompson grapes (3.5 oz)	11	67	0.2		
*Pears Pearldale	39	238	0.2	✓	
*Fettucini Sausalito	85	537	0.2	✓	
*Codfish Blue Lake	15	95	0.2	✓	✓
*Strawberry- Champagne Mold Strawberry Creek	29	191	0.2		
French Bread (3.5 oz)	43	290	0.1		

Albacore (tuna) (3.5 oz)	26	177	0.1	
*Fresh Fruit Fresno	80	575	0.1	
*Spaghettini with Clam Sauce Pismo Beach	80	580	0.1	✓
*Halibut Steak with Capers Capistrano	16	124	0.1	✓
*Fresh Fruit Sorbet Stovepipe Wells	33	256	0.1	✓
Canned tuna (3.5 oz)	16	127	0.1	
*Vermicelli with Sauce San Bruno	74	601	0.1	✓
Apple (3.5 oz)	7	58	0.1	
Pear (3.5 oz)	7	61	0.1	
Chicken Breast (3.5 oz)	11	101	0.1	
White wine (3.5 oz)	9	85	0.1	
*Orange Roughy Oakland	15	143	0.1	
Applesauce, unsweetened (3.5 oz)	4	41	0.1	✓
*Mushrooms & Pasta Mill Valley	57	587	0.1	✓
*Baked Apples Applegate	22	228	0.1	✓
Banana (3.5 oz)	8	85	0.1	
*Sole Marina del Rey	14	152	0.1	✓
*Apple-Cranberry Mold Alpine	15	164	0.1	
*Rice Pilaf Ranchita	8	90	0.1	✓ ✓
*Pasta Fiesta Island	29	339	0.1	✓
*Peaches Paradise Valley	23	307	0.1	

Pasta (3.5 oz)	11	148	0.1	
*Peaches Pacifica	21	283	0.1	✓ ✓
Nectarine (3.5 oz)	4	64	0.1	
*Bananas Santa Barbara	17	281	0.1	✓
*Apple Crumble Julian	18	299	0.1	✓
*Citrus Sorbet San Diego	7	297	0.0	✓ ✓

NOTE: Bok choy is nominally very high in calcium. However, it has not been tested for oxalates, and should be used sparingly until more information is available. Watercress and parsley, which are nominally high in calcium, are high in oxalates.

*See Recipe section for all foods marked with an asterisk.

9

The Low-Calorie Calcium Diet

T he following is a high-calcium, *low-calorie* diet especially for people who want to increase their calcium intake but also want to lose weight. The diet runs for thirty days, and you may repeat the cycle. However, we recommend using it for no longer than two months at a time. The diet contains 60 percent complex carbohydrates, 20 percent protein, and 20 percent fat, including a large amount of omega-3 fish oils. Be sure to take a daily multiple vitamin and mineral supplement that contains at least 18 milligrams of iron and 5 milligrams of manganese, such as Centrum from Lederle.

The diet begins on the weekend, with two "cleansing days" of delicious but extra-low-calorie foods, emphasizing fruits and fluids. For the remaining 28 days the daily plan limits your food intake to 1200 calories. In general, the diet follows the same principles found in the regular Calcium Connection diet in Chapter 8.

The cornerstone of the diet is our own special "La Jolla Shake," easily prepared in the blender from milk, fruit, and tofu.

In general, we suggest no substitutions in the plan. However, if necessary, the foods in each of the following groupings *are* interchangeable:

oranges, bananas, grapes

grapefruit, pears, apples, plums, peaches, nectarines

skim milk, buttermilk

If necessary, after the first two "cleansing" days, you may nibble up to four ounces of the following raw vegetables to satisfy any between-meal hunger pains: cucumber, broccoli, carrots, celery, or cauliflower.

A different menu is presented for each day—no two days are alike. An asterisk (*) next to a dish means that a recipe for it is given in Part III. You are allowed one serving of each dish—sorry, no seconds. If no amount of food is listed, it means that a standard three-and-one-half ounce portion is intended. "Milk" means non-fat milk or buttermilk, eight ounces. We assume eight ounce portions of juice and herb tea also. "Wine" means six ounces of table or vintage wine, not fortified wines such as sherry or port. For vegetables, "hot" means steamed.

DAY 1 / FIRST CLEANSING DAY / SATURDAY

BREAKFAST	**MID-AFTERNOON**
*La Jolla Shake	Spring water
MID-MORNING	**DINNER**
Herb tea	*La Jolla Shake
LUNCH	**EVENING**
*La Jolla Shake	Herb tea or fruit juice

DAY 2 / SECOND CLEANSING DAY / SUNDAY

BREAKFAST	**MID-AFTERNOON**
*La Jolla Shake	Herb tea
MID-MORNING	**DINNER**
Grapefruit juice	*La Jolla Shake
LUNCH	**EVENING**
*La Jolla Shake	Apple juice

DAY 3 / MONDAY / WEEK 1

BREAKFAST
*La Jolla Shake
Raisin toast

LUNCH
Fruit

SNACK
Apple juice

DINNER
*Chicken Breasts Santa
  Ysabel
Hot broccoli with lemon
  wedge
Hot rice
Wine
Fruit (2 servings)

SNACK
Milk (half glass)

DAY 4 / TUESDAY / WEEK 1

BREAKFAST
*La Jolla Shake

LUNCH
Grapes (2 servings)
Roll
Milk

DINNER
*Spaghetti San Francisco

Romaine and cucumber with
  olive oil (2 teaspoons),
  vinegar, and herbs
Bread
Wine
Fruit

SNACK
Fruit

DAY 5 / WEDNESDAY / WEEK 1

BREAKFAST
*La Jolla Shake

LUNCH
Milk
Fruit
Cinnamon bagel (½)

SNACK
Milk (half glass)

DINNER
*Codfish Blue Lake
*Red Cabbage Reseda
Hot new potato with
  margarine
Wine
*Citrus Sorbet San Diego

SNACK
Fruit

DAY 6 / THURSDAY / WEEK 1

BREAKFAST
*La Jolla Shake
Raisin toast

LUNCH
Fruit
Roll
Milk (half glass)

DINNER
*Linguine Lafayette
Wine
Fruit

SNACK
Apple juice

DAY 7 / FRIDAY / WEEK 1

BREAKFAST
*La Jolla Shake

LUNCH
Fruit
Milk

DINNER
*Caesar Salad Coronado
French roll
Wine
*Bananas Santa Barbara

DAY 8 / SATURDAY / WEEK 1

BREAKFAST
*La Jolla Shake

LUNCH
*Stuffed Eggs Escondido
Fruit (2 servings)
*Poppyseed Dressing
  California
Roll

DINNER
*Scallops San Simeon
*Broccoli Bel Air
*Compote Apple Valley
Wine

DAY 9 / SUNDAY / WEEK 1

BREAKFAST
*La Jolla Shake

LUNCH
Pasta salad
Apple juice

DINNER
*Salmon Seacliff
Hot broccoli
Wine
*Fruit Sorbet Rancho
  Santa Fe

DAY 10 / MONDAY / WEEK 2

BREAKFAST
*La Jolla Shake

LUNCH
Fruit
Roll
Grapefruit juice (half glass)

DINNER
*Pasta Shells Siciliano
Cucumber with 1 teaspoon
  olive oil, lemon juice, and
  herbs
Wine

SNACK
Apple juice

DAY 11 / TUESDAY / WEEK 2

BREAKFAST
*La Jolla Shake

LUNCH
Fruit
Roll
Apple juice

DINNER
*Chicken Kabobs Malibu
  Colony
Corn on the cob
Cabbage slaw with lemon
  juice, olive oil, and herbs
Wine
Fruit

SNACK
Milk

DAY 12 / WEDNESDAY / WEEK 2

BREAKFAST
*La Jolla Shake

LUNCH
Grapes
Roll
Milk (half glass)

SNACK
Apple juice

DINNER
*Vegetable Caviar Viola
Bread (2 slices)
Wine
*Citrus Sorbet San Diego

SNACK
Milk (6 ounces)

DAY 13 / THURSDAY / WEEK 2

BREAKFAST
*La Jolla Shake

LUNCH
Fruit
Bread
Milk (half glass)

DINNER
*Broccoli Tierrasanta
Cooked pasta tossed with
    margarine (unsalted)
Tomato slices
Wine
*Peaches Pacifica

SNACK
Apple juice

DAY 14 / FRIDAY / WEEK 2

BREAKFAST
*La Jolla Shake

SNACK
Fruit

LUNCH
Fruit
Roll
Milk

DINNER
*Shrimp with Pasta San Luis
    Rey
Wine
Fruit
*Poppyseed Dressing
    California

DAY 15 / SATURDAY / WEEK 2

BREAKFAST
*La Jolla Shake

LUNCH
*Cream of Champagne Soup
  Cardiff (half serving)
Hot asparagus
*Mayonnaise Malibu

DINNER
*Salmon Mold San Carlos
Romaine with oil, lemon
  juice, and herbs
Wine
*Citrus Sorbet San Diego

DAY 16 / SUNDAY / WEEK 2

BREAKFAST
*La Jolla Shake

SNACK
Fruit

LUNCH
Turkey breast and tomato
  sandwich
Cabbage slaw with lemon
  juice
Fruit
Milk (half glass)

DINNER
*Shrimp Laguna Beach
Cucumber
Wine
*Fruit Sorbet Rancho
  Santa Fe

DAY 17 / MONDAY / WEEK 3

BREAKFAST
*La Jolla Shake

LUNCH
Fruit
Roll
Milk (half glass)

DINNER
*Cheese Log Canoga
Cucumber slices
Roll
Wine
Fruit

SNACK
Fruit

DAY 18 / TUESDAY / WEEK 3

BREAKFAST
*La Jolla Shake

LUNCH
Fruit
Roll
Apple juice

DINNER
*Pasta Penasquitos
Baby turnips
Broccoli
Lemon juice
Wine
*Citrus Sorbet San Diego

DAY 19 / WEDNESDAY / WEEK 3

BREAKFAST
*La Jolla Shake

LUNCH
Fruit
Roll
Milk (half glass)

SNACK
Apple juice

DINNER
*Salmon Sausalito
Hot cabbage
Hot new potatoes
Parmesan cheese (1
   teaspoon)
Wine
Fruit

SNACK
Fruit

DAY 20 / THURSDAY / WEEK 3

BREAKFAST
*La Jolla Shake
Bread

LUNCH
Fruit
Roll
Milk

DINNER
*Vegetable-Yogurt Loaf
   Tecopa
*Rice Pilaf Ranchita
   (2 servings)
Wine
Fruit (2 servings)

SNACK
Apple juice

DAY 21 / FRIDAY / WEEK 3

BREAKFAST
*La Jolla Shake

LUNCH
Fruit
Roll
Apple juice

DINNER
*Lasagna Live Oak
Cucumber slices
Wine

DAY 22 / SATURDAY / WEEK 3

BREAKFAST
*La Jolla Shake

LUNCH
Cucumber, tomato, and
  cooked pasta
*Anchovy Spread Angel's
  Camp
Milk (half glass)

SNACK
Apple juice

DINNER
*Oysters Pirate Cove
Romaine and sliced radishes
  tossed with olive oil, lemon
  juice, and herbs
Champagne
Fruit

SNACK
Fruit

DAY 23 / SUNDAY / WEEK 3

BREAKFAST
*La Jolla Shake

LUNCH
*Eggs Exeter
Fruit
Milk

DINNER
*Chicken Carlsbad
Cabbage slaw with lemon
  juice
Wine
Fruit

SNACK
Fruit

DAY 24 / MONDAY / WEEK 4

BREAKFAST
*La Jolla Shake

LUNCH
Fruit
Roll
Milk (half glass)

DINNER
*Chef's Salad Half Moon Bay
Wine
Fruit
*Fruit Salad Dressing Soledad
   (2 teaspoons)
*Citrus Sorbet San Diego

SNACK
Fruit

DAY 25 / TUESDAY / WEEK 4

BREAKFAST
*La Jolla Shake

LUNCH
Fruit
Roll
Milk (6 ounces)

DINNER
*Fettucine Sunland
Sliced cucumber and tomato
   with olive oil, vinegar, and
   herbs
Wine
*Fruit Sorbet Rancho
   Santa Fe

SNACK
Apple juice

DAY 26 / WEDNESDAY / WEEK 4

BREAKFAST
*La Jolla Shake

LUNCH
Fruit
Roll
Milk

DINNER
*Croquettes Campo
Hot baby carrots
Roll with margarine
Wine
Fruit

SNACK
Apple juice

DAY 27 / THURSDAY / WEEK 4

BREAKFAST
*La Jolla Shake

LUNCH
Fruit
Roll
Grapefruit juice

DINNER
*Salmon Shell Beach
Cooked pasta
Sliced cucumber
Wine
Fruit
*Fruit Sorbet Rancho Santa
  Fe

SNACK
Fruit

DAY 28 / FRIDAY / WEEK 4

BREAKFAST
*La Jolla Shake
Raisin bread

LUNCH
Fruit
Roll
Milk (half glass)

SNACK
Fruit

DINNER
*Omelet Ocotillo
Lettuce and cauliflower with
  lemon juice
Wine
Fruit
*Poppyseed Dressing
  California

SNACK
Fruit

DAY 29 / SATURDAY / WEEK 4

BREAKFAST
*La Jolla Shake

LUNCH
*Shrimp Dip Diamond
  Springs
Cauliflower flowerets
Cucumber spears
Milk

DINNER
Chicken breast grilled with
  lemon juice and herbs

Cooked pasta
Hot cabbage with herbs and
  lemon juice
Wine
*Cherries Chula Vista (½
  serving)

SNACK
Fruit

DAY 30 / SUNDAY / WEEK 4

BREAKFAST
*La Jolla Shake

LUNCH
*Sea Salad Seal Beach
Milk (half glass)
Fruit

DINNER
*Ravioli Riverside
Fruit
Wine

A HIGH-CALCIUM, LACTOSE-FREE, LOW-CALORIE DIET

Some people are unable to digest lactose, making it impossible for them to consume milk and other dairy products. Nonetheless, such people can still have a diet rich in calcium and other nutrients while losing weight. This is possible because some vegetables, fish, and shellfish have two, three, or even four times as much calcium as calories. Some of these foods are broccoli, bok choy, cabbage, onions, artichokes, sardines, and anchovies. Oranges, eastern oysters, cauliflower, and cucumber all have high calcium to calories ratio as well.

The following week-long, high-calcium, low-calorie diet is without lactose. Be sure that in addition you drink two-and-one-half quarts of water each day.

MONDAY

BREAKFAST
Orange sections (2 servings)
Roll

LUNCH
Fruit
Roll

DINNER
Canned salmon (2 servings)
Pasta shells (2 servings)
Broccoli and butterhead
  lettuce
Wine

TUESDAY

BREAKFAST
Orange sections
Rolls (2)

LUNCH
Fruit
*Poppyseed Dressing
  California
*Stuffed Eggs Escondido
  (2 servings)

DINNER
Shrimp steamed with dill and
  lemon
Asparagus
Raw broccoli with lemon
  juice (2 servings)
Wine
Fruit

WEDNESDAY

BREAKFAST
Orange sections (2 servings)
Roll

LUNCH
Lettuce
Tomato
Cucumber and onions
Oil and vinegar
Fruit

DINNER
Sardines in tomato sauce
Rice
Broccoli
Wine
Fruit

THURSDAY

BREAKFAST
Orange sections (2 servings)
Rolls (2)

LUNCH
Hard cooked egg
Lettuce
Tofu cubes
Apple sauce
Tomato
Onion
Lemon juice
Fruit

DINNER
Hot pasta tossed with
　　anchovies, tomato, broccoli
　　and lemon juice
　　(2 servings)
Wine
Fruit

FRIDAY

BREAKFAST
Orange sections (2 servings)
Rolls (2)

LUNCH
Raw broccoli (2 servings)
Bread (1 slice)
Cucumber

DINNER
Grilled salmon (7 ounces)
Hot kale
Wine
Fruit

SATURDAY

BREAKFAST
Orange sections (2 servings)
Rolls (2)

LUNCH
Cabbage slaw (2 servings)
  with lemon juice
Tofu cubes
Pineapple
Thompson grapes
  (2 servings)

DINNER
Shrimp, steamed
Baby peas
Raw broccoli and cauliflower
  with mayonnaise
  (2 servings)
Wine

SUNDAY

BREAKFAST
Orange sections (2 servings)
Rolls (2)

LUNCH
Raw broccoli (2 servings)
Cucumber with lemon juice
Bagel
Apple

DINNER
Eastern oysters (2 servings)
  with hot sauce
Chilled pasta with escarole,
  onion, and lemon juice
Wine
Fruit

10

Supplements

The most frequent question that we are asked after we have given a talk about the benefits of vitamin D and calcium is: What do you recommend as a supplement? We usually answer this with a few questions to the person who asked us, such as whether the person is intolerant of milk.

There are no long-term studies of the effect of supplements on risk of almost any disease. But there are a number of studies on the effect of food. It is clear that food containing vitamin D and calcium reduces risk of certain cancers and other calcium-deficiency related diseases. We use a conservative approach, and recommend that people obtain calcium and vitamin D from natural foods in their diet.

It has been estimated that about 10 percent of the U.S. population has difficulty digesting the natural sugar in milk called lactose. If you can't tolerate lactose, you will have to try alternatives to regular milk. Some people who can't tolerate milk seem to be able to tolerate yogurt. Yogurt is a rich source of calcium (410 milligrams per 8-ounce cup) and will supply the calcium you need. Look for brands that contain only milk and active *Bacillus acidophilis, Bacillus bulgaris* or similar cultures. Avoid brands that contain carrageenan, a chemical that produces an intestinal disease, ulcerative colitis, in animals. Although the FDA allows carrageenan to be used now, we feel its use in foods should be discontinued pending appropriate epidemiologic studies. Eat low-fat yogurt whenever possible.

If you cannot eat yogurt, or simply do not like yogurt, there are other possibilities. Lactose can be removed from milk with lactase enzymes. Milk is now available with much of the lactose removed and you may be able to tolerate it better. If you are trying yogurt or lactose-reduced milk for the first time, begin with a small amount—say a tablespoon or two—working up to larger amounts only if you can tolerate the small ones.

If you try these options, and others, such as fish, tofu, and vegetables containing high usable calcium, as shown in the calcium counter at the back of the book, and still can't get your calcium level to the 800 to 1,200 milligrams recommended per day, you may need a calcium supplement.

There are several criteria you should use in picking a supplement: *Absorption,* or the amount of calcium absorbed per milligram of calcium present in the tablet; *Tolerance,* or how well your body accepts the supplement; *Side effects* (see Chapter 12); *Special situations,* such as existing diseases for which supplements could create problems; *Interactions,* or problems that could occur because you are taking another medicine at the same time as the supplement; and *Cost,* since you don't want to pay more than is necessary for safe, effective supplementation.

Calcium supplements should be taken only after individual evaluation and advice of a doctor or nutritionist, particularly in children or anyone who is bedridden. Children can usually get enough calcium from food alone and do not require calcium supplements, except on the advice of a pediatrician. People who are bedridden usually do not need supplements, since inactivity causes calcium levels in the blood to rise as bone mass drops. Adding calcium can create trouble in such people.

Unfortunately, manufacturers of calcium carbonate tablets and other calcium preparations have yet to show that calcium works as well in the form of tablets as it does in food. Several years ago (1982), an epidemiological study by our colleague Dr. Richard Shekelle and his colleagues in Chicago showed a benefit of vitamin A in preventing cancer of the lung in smokers. Smokers purchased vitamin A pills in hope of achieving similar effect. What they did not know was that the form of vitamin A that had produced the benefit, carotene, was very different from the retinol form that was then being sold over-the-counter in most states. Carotene is a pigment common in nature and has powerful antioxidant properties that prevent various reactions within the body. Retinol is a much poorer antioxidant. The vitamin A people took in the form of supplements probably did them little good, as it was probably the antioxidant properties more than the other characteristics of carotene that provided the protection.

VITAMIN D

The number of foods containing vitamin D is limited. We feel it would be beneficial if the dairy industry added small amounts of vitamin D to yogurt, cottage cheese, and other dairy products in order to provide a range of choices for the consumer. Presently, no dairy products other than milk contain significant amounts of vitamin D year-round.

Perhaps the most common complaint about consumption of foods containing vitamin D is that many of them are high in calories. But by making careful choices, calories can be kept low. Fish, for example, provides vitamin D, as well as the omega-3 fatty acids that protect against heart disease.

Nonfat milk contains large amounts of calcium *and* vitamin D, and there are only 81 calories in an eight-ounce glass (as well as 271 milligrams of calcium).

Use vitamins in moderation. Too many people have a tendency to think they have covered their bases with the latest multivitamin pill and skip foods that might provide such vitamins naturally. Many of the secrets of preventing cancer and other diseases are not yet available in a vitamin bottle. It's true that we live in a pill-oriented age. But the more we resist the notion that a vitamin or other kind of pill will take care of all our needs, the better off we are likely to be. You would accomplish more by choosing a salmon steak for dinner, drinking nonfat milk, eating yogurt and fresh fruit, taking the time to prepare fresh vegetables, exercising, and using *The Calcium Connection* diet in this book.

CALCIUM CARBONATE

At the moment calcium carbonate seems to be the best of the calcium supplements. It provides the largest dose per tablet of calcium of anything available. It doesn't seem to differ much from other calcium supplements in absorbability in healthy adults.

If you drop a calcium carbonate tablet in a glass of water, it will not dissolve. Calcium carbonate is relatively insoluble in ordinary water. Most drinking water, of course, already contains calcium — it is the principal ingredient that makes water hard (it's the white powder left behind in the coffee pot or the saucepan when you boil hard water). If you add some lemon juice or vinegar to the water, however, the calcium carbonate will dissolve. Normally, this is the job your stomach accomplishes when you eat a meal rich in calcium. Eating causes your stomach to release hydrochloric acid, and in an acid medium, the tablet dissolves.

This makes calcium carbonate a good choice if you decide to use supplements and you are healthy. But some people don't have enough hydrochloric acid on tap in their stomach. This deficiency is known as achlorhydria and is common in the elderly. If you lack enough acid, swallowing a calcium carbonate tablet will be almost like dropping it in a glass of plain water. It will not dissolve in your stomach. There is a chance some of it will dissolve elsewhere in your gastrointestinal system, because bacteria can sometimes produce acids that will help aid calcium digestion. But the benefits of taking calcium carbonate will be substantially reduced.

There is another potential drawback to using calcium carbonate supplements. In places throughout the world where sanitation is poor, acid in the stomach provides a barrier against harmful organisms present in food and water. A lot of common organisms that cause disease are killed by acids when they enter the stomach. The acid therefore serves a dual role: it helps digest food, and also reduces the bacterial count and helps to prevent disease. Calcium carbonate tends to *reduce* the acidity of the stomach. When the stomach is neutralized by regular intake of calcium supplements, the acid barrier against bacteria may be weakened. Food and water sanitation is generally excellent in the United States, so the problem here is minimal. But if you travel extensively or live somewhere where food and water sanitation is marginal, you may want to restrict or reduce your calcium carbonate intake.

Calcium carbonate is both the cheapest and the most readily available kind of calcium supplement. It can be found in drug stores and health-food stores in certain over-the-counter products. Check labels carefully.

If you do decide to take calcium carbonate supplements, be careful not to consume them with calcium food robbers, as much of the calcium would be bound up and made unusable.

CALCIUM GLUCONATE

This compound is similar to that of calcium carbonate. Calcium gluconate is made by combining calcium with glucose, the simplest sugar. Calcium gluconate is probably tolerated by most people as well as calcium carbonate.

Calcium gluconate contains only 9 percent elemental calcium.

If you choose this supplement, you will need to take a great many more tablets to get a reasonable amount of calcium. Like calcium carbonate, this supplement is best taken with meals, because calcium in general dissolves better in acid. Calcium gluconate is somewhat more expensive than calcium carbonate, which may affect your choice of supplement.

CALCIUM LACTATE

This preparation contains about 13 percent calcium. With calcium lactate, you don't need to worry about neutralization of stomach acid as much as with calcium carbonate. As with other forms of calcium supplements, calcium lactate is best taken with meals. Again, be careful not to include calcium robbers with your meal, in order to obtain the full benefit from the calcium supplement.

OTHER PREPARATIONS

There are several preparations of calcium that we do not recommend. Bone meal is one. It is made from ground animal bones. Animals are subject to the same pollution that we are and many absorb lead and other pollutants, storing them in their bones. When you consume bone meal you are consuming an animal's lifetime of stored pollutants—not much of a bargain. Oyster shells, too, are pulverized and sold as calcium supplements. Their safety and purity depends upon where the oysters were harvested. If they were from an area contaminated with industrial waste, such as lead, the oyster shells can incorporate the lead and pass it on to you. Dolomite, an ancient chalky compound, may also contain contaminants such as lead and arsenic. We recommend that you avoid these sources of calcium supplementation. It is especially important to avoid them for infants, children, and women who are pregnant or nursing.

Other calcium compounds are sometimes recommended as supplements but none have the safety of calcium carbonate, calcium lactate, and calcium gluconate.

When calcium is consumed in food, it is usually in beverages or foods that are high in water content. Milk is mostly water, and many vegetables have high water content along with calcium. Water ensures that the calcium will be soluble in the stomach and in the intestine so that it can be absorbed. It also prevents the formation of crystals of calcium oxalate, calcium phosphate, and other compounds in the kidneys that can lead to kidney stones. One of the reasons that food is safer than supplements is because of water content. If you must supplement your diet with calcium tablets, be sure to drink at least two-and-one-half quarts of water per day.

Several grocery store items contain added calcium, such as orange or grapefruit drinks found in the dairy case. The producers of these products mean well, but because they are not natural foods—only part fruit juice—the added calcium is not necessarily a good tradeoff. Nonetheless, in terms of calcium, these drinks are safer than supplements, because of the fluid content. In addition, some soft drinks also have added calcium, but the amount is not enough to be beneficial.

11

The Importance of Water

The average American drinks two quarts of water daily. He or she also drinks twelve ounces of soft drinks and eleven ounces of milk a day. The fact is, we can't live without water. Two thirds of the water we consume goes directly into our cells. The rest goes into the bloodstream and the spaces surrounding the cells. All tissues in the body allow water to pass through. No other liquid has this distinction.

Your body is finely tuned to retain a constant concentration of body fluids. It does this very precisely by retaining water in proportion to anything dissolved in the body fluids. When we need to dilute salt or sugar, for example, because the concentration has risen, cells in a part of our brain called the hypothalamus send out a signal. We interpret the signal as thirst. When we dilute the salt and sugar enough, we are no longer thirsty.

It is important with *The Calcium Connection* diet that you drink plenty of water and liquids throughout the day. We recommend at least two-and-one-half quarts per day. Water is essential to a healthy body, and will help you to dissolve and absorb the increased calcium that you take in, whether from food or from supplements.

Although you may not realize it, the dietary substance with the highest calcium-to-calorie ratio is water. Some water contains as much as 200 milligrams of calcium per quart and has no calories. You can take in 400 milligrams of calcium each day without adding any calories by drinking calcium-rich water. Unfortunately, U.S. municipal water contains on the average only 26 milligrams of calcium per quart. Unless you live in a city where the calcium levels are high, you'll have to get most of your daily calcium from the food you eat. If you do live in a city where the calcium level per quart of water approaches 200 milligrams, however, you may be able, by drinking two quarts or more a day, to obtain over one third of our recommended daily calcium intake from water alone.

If you're worried about taking in too much calcium because your city water supply is high in calcium, rest assured that there is no danger. According to the National Academy of Sciences, there has never been a report of acute toxicity from consumption of the calcium contained in ordinary amounts of food or drinking water. Drink as much water as you like. In fact, it is unwise to take in large amounts of calcium *without* also taking in lots of fluids, because calcium can't be absorbed well or excreted safely without water. Fluids are excellent vehicles for calcium.

Drinking water with high levels of calcium can also help in other ways. A high intake of calcium decreases absorption of lead and other toxic trace metals from the intestine. It has been shown that the amount of calcium in the blood is inversely related to the amount of lead.

Calcium also prevents intestinal absorption of cadmium, a trace metal that can cause serious diseases. Cadmium can make the body produce lower than usual levels of vitamin D, which is important for active absorption of calcium. This creates a vicious cycle leading to still less absorption of calcium and eventually to bone damage.

According to the National Academy of Sciences, "No upper limit for calcium in drinking water needs to be set to protect public health. In cases of calcium deficiencies, the presence of this element in drinking water provides nutritional benefit."

BOTTLED WATER

Almost all bottled waters are bacteriologically pure. Because of that, purity is not a significant factor in choosing a bottled water. In that sense, it doesn't matter *where* a water is from, since there is no reason to believe that water from one state or country, such as Arkansas or France, is any different structurally from water anywhere else. What does differ is the chemical content of the water.

There are three types of bottled water used for drinking. The first is distilled or deionized water, which is water from which all the elements have been removed by boiling or putting it through a device known as a deionizer. It is not wise to consume distilled or deionized water on a daily basis because it contains no trace calcium or other minerals.

The second kind of water used for drinking is spring water, or "drinking water." Spring water comes out of the earth on its own pressure without piping, although a short pipe is permitted in the spring. If the water doesn't come out of the ground on its own, it is not spring water. Such water is usually called well water, although it is sometimes called "mountain" or "natural" water. The term "drinking water" is also widely used, but has no meaning. It can apply to anything from deionized or distilled water, spring or well water, to municipal water that may have been deionized.

Finally there is mineral water. In California, mineral water must contain at least 500 parts per million of dissolved solids, but it is not regulated this way in most of the United States. Mineral water may contain large amounts of sodium, since sodium content is not subject to meaningful restrictions. People with high blood pressure should avoid mineral water unless they know it is low in sodium.

Because the calcium content in bottled water is rarely provided on the label, it is usually impossible to know how much calcium you may be getting from water if you consume bottled water on a daily basis.

THE DIFFERENCES IN MUNICIPAL WATER

Water varies drastically from region to region. The variations in water in different cities *are* important. The water supply in San Diego, California, for example, contains 67 milligrams of calcium per quart, while the water supply in San Francisco contains none. (You can look up the calcium and magnesium content of the water in your city in Appendix B). A person drinking San Diego water takes in 134 milligrams more calcium from water alone each day than a person drinking San Francisco water. This 134 milligrams a day can be the difference between positive and negative calcium balance.

If your city water supply is low in calcium, you'll have to make special efforts to be sure to get enough calcium from your diet. Unfortunately, most bottled waters, whether mineral or spring water, do not list the calcium content in them. So if you drink bottled water primarily, you'll have no way of knowing how much calcium you're getting from the water. To ensure that you get enough calcium daily, assume that the spring water you drink has no calcium, and gauge your daily calcium intake from the foods you eat.

HARD WATER

Hard water refers to water with high concentrations of calcium and magnesium. We have now learned that hard water can have health benefits. According to a report from the National Academy of Sciences in 1979, studies of large geographic areas have found that hard water is linked with low rates of heart disease. The scientific panel reported that drinking soft water might increase risk of heart disease by as much as 25 percent, and risk of stroke and hypertension by as much as 20 percent.

The epidemiological evidence strongly suggests that soft water is not as healthy as hard water. We are surprised when we hear that a public water supply system is softening its water, because the methods used for water softening cut water's calcium content and usually raise the sodium content. The likely result: a slightly increased risk of hypertension, heart disease, and stroke in people who drink the water.

Home water softeners are just as bad in terms of health. Most home water softeners remove one atom of calcium or magnesium and replace it with two atoms of sodium. It's an unwise practice.

THE DANGER OF ALUMINUM

One of the chemicals found in the water you drink is aluminum. High doses of aluminum can interfere with absorption of calcium. Until 1974 aluminum was regarded as a nontoxic material. Recent studies have changed that viewpoint. Aluminum is found in unusually high concentrations in the tissues of the nervous system of people who have Alzheimer's Disease. We don't know whether this is due to buildup of aluminum from water or foods, but it is a finding that has stirred considerable interest.

Why is aluminum so dangerous? Like calcium, aluminum is a positively charged ion—a cation. Like calcium it is a metal. When tissues in your body need calcium, they send out an SOS informing the body. When the need can't be met by calcium, the hungry cells absorb aluminum instead.

People on kidney dialysis absorb aluminum from water entering dialysis machines and sometimes develop aluminum poisoning. This causes a type of dementia very similar to Alzheimer's Disease, and is the leading cause of death in longtime dialysis patients.

When the Chicago water department added aluminum to part of the public water supply, thirteen patients in a local dialysis clinic soon developed dementia. Doctors at the clinic said they had not seen the problem before the aluminum was added. Before the city water department began adding aluminum, the water contained about 75 micrograms of aluminum per quart. When the aluminum was added, the concentration climbed to 350 micrograms per quart, a fivefold increase. The aluminum was added in the form of aluminum sulfate, a water-treatment compound.

12

Side Effects

No discussion of a program to increase dietary calcium is complete without consideration of possible side effects and how you can minimize them. Fortunately, the side effects of calcium are almost nonexistent at levels found in the normal diet. But the side effects of large overdoses of vitamin D can be serious.

The U.S. Department of Agriculture estimates that adult men in the United States consume an average of 724 milligrams of calcium per day. Women take in about two-thirds that amount. We take in about 10 percent less if we live in cities, about 10 percent more if we live in farming areas. Some people consume 2,000 milligrams of calcium per day with no apparent toxicity or side effects.

People who treat their own indigestion or ulcers by taking large amounts of antacids, some of which are high in calcium compounds, may develop *milk-alkali syndrome,* which deposits calcium in unusual places in the body. This is uncommon, however, and is usually readily reversed by cutting down on antacids. But the risk of developing the syndrome is virtually nonexistent for those who obtain calcium from ordinary foods and beverages. It is, however, one reason we do not recommend calcium supplements. If you are taking antacids on your own advice, or on the advice of your doctor, consult your doctor before adding additional calcium to your diet.

The daily intakes of calcium shown in the tables on pages 82–83 should not be exceeded. These recommendations are in general similar to those of the National Academy of Sciences, with corrections for people living in areas of low ultraviolet light.

Your body very carefully regulates its absorption of calcium. If you take in too much, the intestine will absorb less. On the average, only about 15 to 35 percent of the calcium we consume is absorbed (partly because much of the calcium we consume is bound to chemical compounds which make it unusable). If your body is deficient in calcium, the intestine tries to compensate, absorbing more.

VITAMIN D

It is impossible to get an overdose of vitamin D from exposure to the sun, although with excessive exposure you *can* cause sunburn, and raise your risk of skin cancer. It is also almost impossible to get an overdose of vitamin D from milk or other sources in the diet.

It is, however, possible to get too much vitamin D from vitamin supplements. People have been known to take in 50,000 IU or more of vitamin D per day. While large doses such as this can sometimes be administered safely under the close supervision of a doctor for treatment of specific medical problems, taken by a healthy person, such large doses can increase the body's demand for calcium beyond what an ordinary diet can provide. The result depends upon the degree of overdose. An excessive amount of vitamin D can lead to hypercalcification or excessive deposition of calcium throughout the body, including the kidneys, as well as excessive loss of calcium from bone, the opposite effect of what is produced by ordinary dietary vitamin D sources.

The effects of vitamin D are especially strong in infants and children. The recommended daily allowance of vitamin D is 400 IU for children and young adults through age eighteen, 300 IU at ages nineteen to twenty-two, and 200 IU at ages twenty-three and older, with an additional 200 IU during pregnancy and breast feeding. *The dose for children should never be exceeded.* For most adults, there is a larger margin of safety, and the restriction on intake need not be as rigid. Adults eighteen years old and older can take in vitamin D from ordinary foods in any reasonable amount with minimal risk. But we do not advise that any healthy person supplement his or her diet with vitamin D in pill or other concentrated forms, except for the amount found in a single ordinary multiple vitamin tablet per day. We strongly caution against the use of any vitamin D supplementation in infants or in pregnant or lactating women. If such supplementation is used, it is very important that the daily dose from all sources not exceed 400 IU in infants and 600 IU in pregnant or lactating women.

Occasionally some individuals are hypersensitive to vitamin D and subject to some toxicity, even at lower dosages. These effects appear to be reversible. Severe cases of infantile hypercalcemia have occurred due to excessive vitamin D supplementation, including some cases possibly induced in utero by excessive supplementary vitamin D taken by the mother. Such excessive supplementation of vitamin D from pills and capsules can induce a syndrome in infants that includes low birth weight and mental, cardiovascular, and renal complications. For this reason we do not recommend any form of supplementation of vitamin D except for supplementation in ordinary foods. We particularly recommend that pregnant women and children not receive vitamin D supplementation other than in foods, and only in special cases.

KIDNEY STONES

The cause of kidney stones is still largely unknown. People with infections, various diseases, certain genetic defects, and dehydration are at particular risk. Most kidney stones contain at least some calcium, but dietary intake of calcium has not been shown conclusively to play a role in causing them. As a precaution, doctors usually limit patients with a history of kidney stones (and in some cases patients with a family history of them) to no more than 400 milligrams per day of calcium. This limitation is the subject of considerable controversy since calcium deficiency may result. Patients are also prohibited from drinking vitamin D-fortified milk or eating other foods rich in vitamin D.

Seventy-five percent of kidney stones in patients in the United States also contain oxalates. There is no standard diet for the reduction of oxalates, but tables are available showing the amount of oxalates in foods (see Appendix E). Most experts on kidney stones believe that it is not calcium intake that causes kidney stones, but rather excess oxalates in the urine that combine with calcium to create the stone.

Excess oxalates in some people may be simply a result of their metabolism. Because of their genetic makeup, they produce more oxalates in the urine, increasing their risk of kidney stones. At this point, it may be impossible to do much about genetically caused excess. But other people have high levels of oxalates in urine because they consume too many foods that are rich in oxalates.

Sources of dietary oxalates for people who have formed stones, or who have a family history of them, should not exceed 40 to 50 milligrams per day.

A surprisingly varied number of foods contain high concentrations of oxalates. Swiss chard, spinach, rhubarb, and even tea are examples. Further information on oxalates in the diet is available in a book by D.M. Ney and associates, entitled *The Low Oxalate Diet Book for the Prevention of Oxalate Kidney Stones,* published by the University of California, San Diego. If you have had kidney stones or have a family history of them, consult your doctor before making any changes in your diet with regard to either oxalates or calcium.

RARE DISEASES

There are a few rare diseases for which calcium intake should be restricted. One example is a skin disease called pseudoxanthoma elasticum. Some scientists have hypothesized that lowering dietary calcium in people with this rare disease might minimize clinical effects. If you have this disease, your calcium intake should be carefully monitored in conjunction with your doctor. Another such disease is sarcoidosis, a relatively uncommon disease that affects various body organs and which can result in overly high levels of calcium in the blood. Another disease where calcium intake must be closely monitored is primary hypercalciuria, which is excessive urinary excretion of calcium. People who have this disease should consult their doctor before altering their calcium or vitamin D intake.

We also advise any patients who are on kidney dialysis to consult with their doctor about their calcium intake, since dialysis interferes with ordinary metabolism of calcium.

We have located one report of a two-year-old girl with pure calcium carbonate gallstones, possibly related to the calcium carbonate supplement her mother took during the last four months of pregnancy. The scientists who reported this stated that they knew of no other such reports. Pregnant women who take calcium supplements should discuss their intake with their obstetricians.

A study by Craig L. Stemmar and associates at the University of Miami Medical School in Florida showed that use of antacids containing magnesium hydroxide and aluminum hydroxide results in a tenfold increase in alkalinity of urine. Because calcium may form stones more readily in alkaline urine, large intakes of such antacids are unwise.

OTHER SIDE EFFECTS

Calcium carbonate tends to reduce the acidity of the stomach. Many people take calcium carbonate as an antacid. Millions of people seem to be able to take calcium carbonate tablets without complications. But such users have probably had excessive acid in the stomach that may have splashed into the esophagus. The tablets may have briefly neutralized some of the acid. For people who do *not* have excessive stomach acid, routine consumption of calcium carbonate could overly neutralize stomach contents. The effects of such neutralization are not known.

One last cautionary note concerns medication for ulcers. Cimetidine is one of the most widely prescribed drugs in the United States. It helps cure ulcers by interfering with gastric secretion. If you are on this or other drugs that produce similar effects, you may not have enough acid in your stomach to dissolve calcium carbonate tablets, particularly if you take them between meals. For such people we recommend increasing calcium intake only through dietary calcium in foods and milk.

13

A Final Note

Y ou are the key to the success of this book. *The Calcium Connection* program will help you to achieve a longer, healthier life—but only if you follow the guidelines the program provides for increasing your calcium intake safely. There is no magic involved. If your diet has been calcium-deficient for twenty years, and you begin to suffer the effects of osteoporosis, increasing your dietary calcium will not suddenly reverse the osteoporosis that has taken so many years to develop. The same is true for cancer. To benefit from *The Calcium Connection* program and diet, you must begin *now*.

It is a program that should last for the rest of your life. But it is not a difficult program to follow. All that we ask is that you eat fresh, good-tasting food—foods that are high in natural calcium—and avoid those few foods that would deplete your calcium supply. The rewards are many.

Establishing a new routine is a challenge. How great the challenge is, and how well you will be able to cope with it, depends on how strongly you're motivated. Decide now that you are going to make a habit of the program outlined in this book. Once you've followed the program for a month or two, you'll find that being careful to eat enough calcium-rich foods will become second nature. After all, a longer, healthier life is certainly worth the effort.

Proper dietary levels of calcium and vitamin D will cut your risk of death from breast and intestinal cancers, and, by following the program now, cut your risk of osteoporosis.

A proper dietary intake of calcium will also bring your blood pressure down a few points. As your blood pressure drops, your risk of heart disease—the number one cause of death in the United States—will be lowered. The diet's low level of saturated fat will also cut your risk of heart disease and you'll decrease your risk of stroke, another prime cause of death in older adults. The risk will be cut even more by the high level of potassium from fresh fruits and vegetables in the diet, which also helps reduce the risk of stroke.

It is a fact that people in countries where large amounts of vitamin D and calcium are consumed tend to have long average life spans. The Japanese, for example, have the highest level of dietary vitamin D in the world; they also have the longest life span. Life expectancy in Japanese men is seventy-three years, and seventy-eight years in women. High levels of consumption of vitamin D from foods alone are consistent with a long life span.

Begin your road to health and longevity by starting *The Calcium Connection* diet now.

PART III
THE
CALCIUM
CONNECTION
RECIPES

The following are the recipes for the starred dishes listed in the calcium diet in Chapter 8 and the calcium-rich weight-loss diet in Chapter 9. We have also included some additional recipes for variety. Each recipe yields four servings.

ALBACORE PARMESAN ALHAMBRA

1 tablespoon olive oil
1 pound albacore tuna fillets
¼ cup dry white wine
½ medium onion, chopped
1 bay leaf, crushed
⅛ teaspoon pepper
1 teaspoon tarragon

Preheat oven to 350 F. Use a 1½-quart shallow casserole. Rub casserole with oil, lay fish on bottom, and pour wine over it. Sprinkle other ingredients on top. Cover and bake for 30 minutes.

ANCHOVY SPREAD ANGEL'S CAMP

1½ cups plain low-fat yogurt
1 tablespoon green onion, chopped fine
1 teaspoon paprika
2-ounce can anchovy fillets
½ teaspoon caraway seed
Pepper
1 teaspoon capers

Beat together (or process in a food processor) all ingredients except capers. Stir in capers. Pack into a crock or bowl, and refrigerate for 2 to 4 hours to blend flavors. Serve on French bread or mix with pasta and vegetables.

Note: For a higher calcium variation, see Anchovy Spread Avalon.

ANCHOVY SPREAD AVALON

> 1½ cups plain low-fat yogurt
> 1 tablespoon green onion, chopped fine
> 1 teaspoon paprika
> 2-ounce can anchovy fillets
> ½ teaspoon caraway seed
> Pepper
> 10 ounces tofu
> 1 teaspoon capers

Beat together (or process in a food processor) all ingredients except capers. Stir in capers. Pack into a crock or bowl, and refrigerate for 2 to 4 hours to blend flavors. Serve on French bread or mix with pasta and vegetables.

APPLE-CRANBERRY MOLD ALPINE

> 1 envelope unflavored gelatin
> 1½ cups plus 2 teaspoons cold water
> ½ cup fructose
> 2 cups fresh cranberries
> 1 cup apples, skinned and diced

Soften the gelatin in 2 teaspoons of cold water. In a large saucepan, combine 1½ cups water with the fructose and bring to a boil. Add cranberries and simmer for 20 minutes. Remove from heat and stir in the gelatin until dissolved. Cool the mixture and add apples. Pour into 1½-quart mold, then chill. Remove from the mold and serve on a cold plate.

APPLE CRUMBLE JULIAN

> 4 medium cooking apples
> 1 teaspoon cinnamon
> ½ cup water

½ cup fructose
½ cup enriched flour
¼ cup safflower margarine

Preheat oven to 375 F. Peel and core the apples, and cut them crosswise in ½-inch thick slices. Arrange the slices in a nonstick casserole, and sprinkle with cinnamon. Add the water.

Work together the fructose, flour, and margarine, creating a crumbly mixture. Spread this over the apples. Bake uncovered for 45 minutes. Serve warm.

Optional: Top with small scoops of sorbet.

BAKED APPLES APPLEGATE

4 large apples
1 cup water
½ lemon, peeled
1 tablespoon raisins
½ cup fructose
¼ cup clover honey
1 teaspoon cinnamon
1 cup water

Core (but do not peel) the apples, taking care not to pierce the bottoms. Remove the top quarter of each apple. Place the apples in a baking dish. Add the water to the dish.

Cut the lemon into small fragments of pulp, and combine with the raisins and half the fructose. Spoon this mixture into the apple cavities.

Preheat the oven to 350 F. Mix the honey, water, cinnamon, and remaining fructose in a sauce pan and boil for 4 minutes. Spoon this mixture over the apples. Bake until tender, for about one hour.

BANANAS SANTA BARBARA

4 tablespoons safflower margarine
4 tablespoons fructose
3 firm yellow (or red) bananas
4 tablespoons California sherry
6 ounces orange juice

Melt the margarine in a chafing dish. Add fructose. Then add bananas sliced lengthwise, cooking until slightly browned. Pour in the sherry and orange juice. Simmer for 10 minutes in liquid. Serve hot, pouring the sauce over the fruit.

BLACKBERRY PUDDING BAY BRIDGE

2 pints of blackberries
1 cup water
6 pieces of day-old white bread, crusts removed
6 tablespoons blackberry wine

Stew the blackberries in water by bringing to a boil and simmering 3 to 4 minutes. Let cool.

Break the bread into chunks and line the bottom of a ceramic casserole with them. Cover the bread with part of the stewed blackberries. Continue making alternate layers until dish is filled. Chill in refrigerator overnight. Serve with blackberry wine spooned over the top.

BLUEBERRY BUNS BASS LAKE

1¼ cups nonfat milk
¼ cup sugar
3 tablespoons clover honey
¼ cup safflower oil
2 packages yeast
¼ cup water, lukewarm
3½ cups enriched flour
3 cups fresh blueberries
¼ cup melted butter

Scald the milk and combine with honey and safflower oil. Cool until lukewarm. Soften yeast in a large bowl of water. Add the lukewarm milk mixture and stir in enough flour to make the dough stiff. Turn the dough onto a lightly floured surface and knead until smooth. Set dough in a greased bowl and brush oil over surface. Cover with a towel and put in a warm place until dough doubles in size (about one hour). Spread the dough out on unfloured surface. Divide in half and roll each half into a rectangle, about ¼-inch thick and 10 inches long. Brush with milk.

Mix the sugar and blueberries together gently. Sprinkle half the mixture on each half of dough. Roll each section gently as if to make a jelly roll. Cut the rolls into ten equal portions. Place on greased baking pans. Brush with melted butter. Cover with waxed paper and let rise for one hour.

Preheat oven to 350 F. Bake 30 minutes. Serve with Whipped Delight Whittier for a special touch.

BAKED BROCCOLI BEL AIR

3 bouquets of broccoli, medium-sized (approximately 1 pound)
Safflower margarine
Dash of pepper
Juice of 1 lemon
2 tablespoons olive oil
3 tablespoons parmesan cheese

Preheat oven to 350 F. Cut broccoli spears into flowerets. Lay in casserole dish greased with safflower margarine. Mix all other ingredients and spread over top. Bake for 30 minutes.

Note: For a higher calcium variation, see Broccoli Berkeley.

BROCCOLI BERKELEY

6 medium-sized bouquets of broccoli (approximately 2 pounds)
Safflower margarine
Dash of pepper
Juice of 1 lemon
4 tablespoons corn oil
1 tablespoon Dijon mustard
6 tablespoons parmesan cheese

Preheat oven to 350 F. Cut broccoli spears into flowerets. Lay in casserole dish greased with safflower margarine. Mix all other ingredients and spread over top. Bake for 30 minutes.

BROCCOLI SOUP BALBOA

1 pound broccoli
2 cloves garlic, minced
6 cups water
1 fresh tomato, cubed
¼ pound spaghetti, broken into 2-inch sections
Pepper
2 tablespoons olive oil
½ cup grated parmesan cheese

Wash and drain broccoli. Soak for 20 minutes in cool water. Cut into inch-size flowerets. Put in pan with garlic, water, and tomato. Bring to a boil over a high flame, then simmer for 10 minutes. Add pasta and sprinkle with pepper. Cook for 15 more minutes, stirring occasionally, or until "al dente." Spoon olive oil over top. Cook 3 minutes longer. Sprinkle grated parmesan cheese on top.

BROCCOLI TIERRASANTA

5 ounces tofu
2 tablespoons virgin olive oil
4 tablespoons parmesan cheese
1 teaspoon dry mustard
1 teaspoon lemon juice
1 clove of garlic, pressed
1 pound broccoli

Stir tofu, oil, cheese, mustard, lemon juice, and garlic together. Place in a double boiler and blend with a whisk while warming. Trim the broccoli flowerets from the stems and steam until tender. Drain and serve immediately topped with the warm sauce.

CAESAR SALAD CORONADO

1 clove garlic
2 ounces olive oil
2 heads romaine lettuce
1 head leaf lettuce, such as Boston or red leaf
Pepper

1 egg
Juice of 2 lemons
16–20 drops Worcestershire sauce
1 tablespoon parmesan cheese, grated
½ cup croutons

Dice garlic and place in oil for several hours.

Tear romaine and lettuce into a salad bowl. Pour the garlic-olive oil mixture over it. Sprinkle fresh ground pepper on top and toss gently once or twice.

Coddle the egg (boil for 1 minute). Break the egg into a bowl and whip lightly with lemon juice and Worcestershire sauce. Add to salad while tossing 2 to 3 times. Sprinkle cheese and croutons over top and toss lightly.

Note: For a higher calcium version variation, see Caesar Salad Salinas.

CAESAR SALAD SALINAS

1 clove garlic
2 ounces olive oil
2 heads romaine
1 head leaf lettuce, such as Boston or red leaf
Pepper
3½ ounces parmesan cheese, grated
1 egg
Juice of 2 lemons
16–20 drops Worcestershire sauce
½ cup croutons
3 anchovies (optional)

Dice garlic and place in oil for several hours.

Tear romaine and lettuce into salad bowl. Pour the garlic-olive oil mixture over it. Sprinkle fresh ground pepper on top and toss gently once or twice.

Coddle the egg (boil for 1 minute). Break the egg into a bowl and whip lightly with lemon juice and Worcestershire sauce. Add to salad while tossing 2 to 3 times. Sprinkle cheese and croutons over top and toss lightly. Top with thin strips of anchovy.

CAULIFLOWER WITH CRAB CARMEL

1 medium head cauliflower
1 can crab bisque
½ cup yogurt
1 tablespoon dry mustard
Dash of pepper

Break cauliflower into flowerets. Steam for 10 minutes or microwave for 2 to 3 minutes. Heat the soup until hot, but not boiling, then stir in the yogurt. Add dry mustard and pepper. Stir mixture over cauliflower.

CHEESE LOG CANOGA

1 pound low-fat cottage cheese
4 ounces blue cheese
4-ounce jar cheddar cheese spread
1 teaspoon Worcestershire sauce
¼ teaspoon onion juice
Pinch of paprika
2 cucumbers

Mix the three cheeses, Worcestershire sauce, and onion juice together. On wax paper shape the mixture into a long roll or ball. Roll in paprika. Chill overnight. Serve on cucumber slices.

CHEESE DIP DEL MAR

10-ounce package silken/soft tofu, well drained
⅛ cup olive oil
2 scallions, sliced thin
2 tablespoons ricotta
1 tablespoon parmesan cheese
Juice of 1 lemon

Beat tofu in mixer or by hand until firm. Stir in remaining ingredients. Chill 2 hours.

Serve with salt-free crackers and raw fresh vegetables, such as carrot sticks, cauliflower and broccoli flowerets, cherry tomatoes.

CHEF'S SALAD CARNELIAN BAY

8 ounces plain low-fat yogurt
2 teaspoons dill seed
4 hard rolls
3 heads romaine lettuce
6-ounce can of unsalted tuna, drained
2 medium tomatoes
4 ounces unsalted (or low-salt) sliced turkey breast

Combine the yogurt and dill seed, and allow the flavors to mature.
Warm the rolls in the oven.

Wash and drain the greens, tear into large pieces, and place in four serving bowls. Flake the tuna onto the lettuce and toss. Cut the turkey breast into thin strips, and arrange on top of the lettuce. Cut the tomatoes into wedges and place on top of the other ingredients.

Add the dill seed dressing, or serve it separately. Serve the rolls along with the salad.

Note: For higher calcium variations, see Chef's Salad Half Moon Bay and Chef's Salad Loma Linda.

CHEF'S SALAD HALF MOON BAY

4 ounces plain low-fat yogurt
2 teaspoons curry powder
4 hard rolls
3 heads romaine lettuce
6-ounce can of unsalted tuna, drained
1 slice Swiss cheese
4 ounces unsalted (or low-salt) sliced turkey breast
2 medium tomatoes

Combine the yogurt and curry powder, and allow the flavors to mature.

Warm the rolls in the oven.

Wash and drain the greens, tear into large pieces, and place in four serving bowls. Flake the tuna onto the lettuce and toss. Slice the cheese and turkey breast into thin strips, and arrange on top of the lettuce. Cut the tomatoes into wedges and place on top of the other ingredients.

Add the curried yogurt dressing, or serve it separately. Serve the rolls along with the salad.

Note: For a higher calcium variation, see Chef's Salad Loma Linda.

CHEF'S SALAD LOMA LINDA

8 ounces plain low-fat yogurt
2 tablespoons lemon juice
4 hard rolls
3 heads romaine
1 6-ounce can of unsalted tuna, drained
2 medium tomatoes
4 slices Swiss cheese
4 ounces unsalted (or low-salt) sliced turkey breast

Combine the yogurt and lemon juice and allow the flavors to mature.

Warm the rolls in the oven.

Wash and drain the greens, tear into large pieces, and place in four serving bowls. Flake the tuna onto the lettuce and toss. Slice the cheese and turkey breast into thin strips, and arrange on top of the lettuce. Cut the tomatoes into wedges and place on top of the other ingredients.

Add the lemon yogurt dressing, or serve it separately. Serve the rolls along with the salad.

CHERRIES CHULA VISTA

1 tablespoon fructose
1 tablespoon cornstarch
2 cups water
1 teaspoon lemon juice
1 pound fresh cherries, pitted and whole
2 cups small pieces of orange (without peels)
1 pint lemon sorbet
½ cup warm brandy

In a cold saucepan, combine the fructose, corn starch, and 1 cup of water, stirring briskly until the cornstarch is dissolved. Bring to a boil and cook until thickened. Add the lemon juice, cherries, and oranges. Simmer until the cherries are tender, adding additional water, if needed.

Serve over the lemon sorbet and top with warm brandy.

CHICKEN BREASTS CATALINA

3 cups fresh mushrooms, about 8 ounces
½ cup 2% milk
1 cup water
Pinch of oregano
Pinch of basil
1 teaspoon margarine
4 skinless chicken breasts

Preheat oven to 350 F. Combine mushrooms, milk, and water in a skillet. Add oregano, basil, and margarine. Cover and simmer for 10 minutes, stirring occasionally.

Place chicken breasts in a square baking pan. Cover each piece with one quarter of the mushroom mixture. Bake 1 hour, or until tender.

Note: For a higher calcium version of this recipe, see Chicken Breasts Santa Ysabel.

CHICKEN BREASTS SANTA YSABEL

3 cups fresh mushrooms, about 8 ounces
½ cup 2% milk
1 cup spring water
Pinch of oregano
Pinch of basil
1 teaspoon margarine
4 skinless chicken breasts
¼ cup parmesan cheese

Preheat oven to 350 F. Combine mushrooms, milk, and water in a skillet. Add oregano, basil, and margarine. Cover and simmer for 10 minutes, stirring occasionally.

Place chicken breasts in a square baking pan. Cover each piece with one quarter of the mushroom mixture. Sprinkle with cheese. Bake 1 hour, or until tender.

CHICKEN CARLSBAD

    4 tablespoons olive oil
    4 chicken breasts, boned and skinned
    Powdered ginger
    Rosemary
    8 ounce plain low-fat yogurt

Rub olive oil on chicken breasts. Sprinkle lavishly with ginger and sparingly with rosemary. Place in shallow baking dish and cover with yogurt. Refrigerate 1 to 2 hours. Broil until golden crust is visible, about 7 minutes. Bake at 350 F uncovered for 50 minutes.

CHICKEN CHEDDAR CASSEROLE CHICO

    4 chicken breasts, about 2 pounds
    2 tablespoons margarine
    1 tablespoon flour
    1 cup nonfat milk
    4 ounces cheddar cheese, grated
    14 ounces broccoli flowerets
    Pinch of thyme
    Pinch of sage

Preheat oven to 350 F. Wrap chicken in foil, place on a baking sheet, and bake about 1 hour.

    Melt margarine in 1-quart saucepan, and make a roux with the flour. Stir in milk and cheese, and continue stirring until thick. Grease the bottom of a 1½-quart casserole. Add broccoli. Remove chicken from oven, place on top of broccoli, and pour sauce over the top. Bake for 20 minutes. Sprinkle with herbs before serving.

CHICKEN KABOBS MALIBU COLONY

    4 large chicken breasts, boneless
    2 teaspoons apple vinegar
    ¼ teaspoon cardamom
    1 tablespoon lemon juice
    2 tablespoons poultry seasoning

2 tablespoons sweet basil, finely ground
2 tablespoons sweet anise
6 tomatoes, skinned and cut in small chunks
10 slices of sweet white onion

Cut breasts into 12 square sections. Turn them in a mixture of vinegar, herbs, and lemon juice. Slide chunks of chicken on wooden skewers alongside tomato chunks and sliced onion. Place under broiler, turning occasionally, for about 15 minutes.

CHICKEN PARMESAN PETALUMA

½ cup bread crumbs, seasoned with 1 teaspoon sage, 1 teaspoon thyme, 1 teaspoon marjoram, pinch of basil, dash of oregano
½ cup parmesan cheese, grated
1 clove of garlic, minced in garlic press
2 tablespoons corn oil
4 chicken breasts

Preheat oven to 350 F. Combine bread crumbs and cheese. Mix garlic into oil. Dip chicken in oil mixture, then roll in crumb mixture. Place on baking pan so that pieces are not touching. Bake 1 hour, or until tender.

CHICKPEAS CALICO

2 cups chickpeas
6 cups water
1 tablespoon olive oil
2 stalks of celery hearts, cut fine
2 green onions (complete), minced fine
Dash of pepper

Wash and soak chickpeas overnight. Boil for 3 hours or until soft, but not mushy. Drain. Heat oil in skillet. Saute celery and onions. Toss with dash of pepper. Stir in the chickpeas and serve at once.

CITRUS SORBET SAN DIEGO

2 cups fructose
4 cups water
¾ cup lime, pink grapefruit, or other citrus juice

Combine fructose and water and boil for 5 minutes. Add citrus juice. Cool, place in a plastic container and freeze. Serve with thin circles of peeled lime on top.

CLAMS ITALIANO

2 tablespoons olive oil
1 clove garlic, mashed
½ white onion, chopped fine
4-ounce can tomato sauce
1 can tomato paste
1 cup water
6-ounce can chopped Chesapeake Bay clams (select type with no additives)
2 salt-free small pizza size crackers*

Heat oil in saucepan. Add garlic and onion and saute until onion is tender. Pour tomato sauce and tomato paste into pan. Add water. Simmer for 15 minutes. Add clams and simmer 15 minutes more. Serve with crackers.

(For lunches, refrigerate sauce and pour into luncheon container.)

CODFISH BLUE LAKE

4 cod fillets, about 1 pound
1 tablespoon olive oil
Juice of 1 lemon
2 cloves of garlic
1 teaspoon pepper
Dash of tarragon
Lemon wedges

*Valley Lahvosh of Fresno, California, makes a select Luncheon-Size Low Sodium cracker.

Preheat the broiler. Rinse fish under cold water and dry with paper towels. Make a paste of the oil, lemon juice, garlic, pepper, and tarragon, and spread on the fish. Broil 3 to 5 minutes on each side. Serve with lemon wedges.

COMPOTE APPLE VALLEY

    4 apples, sliced thin
    3 teaspoons clover honey
    ½ cup water
    3 ounces tofu, cut into ½-inch squares
    1 teaspoon lemon juice
    ¼ teaspoon cinnamon
    1 small lemon, sliced into ornamental crescents

Mix apples, honey, and water thoroughly in a saucepan. Add the tofu gently and cook over a low flame. Cool. Spread lemon juice over the top, then sprinkle on the cinnamon. Chill. Serve with crescents of lemon on the side.

CREAM OF CHAMPAGNE SOUP CARDIFF

    2 tablespoons margarine
    1 large yellow onion, chopped
    1 tablespoon flour
    12 ounces evaporated nonfat milk
    3 cups nonfat milk
    ½ pound broccoli
    ½ pound cauliflower
    4 tablespoons California champagne
    1 teaspoon basil
    1 teaspoon oregano

Melt the margarine in a large saucepan and saute the onion until brown and tender. Sprinkle with flour and stir until dissolved. Gently add the evaporated milk and nonfat milk, stirring constantly over a low flame. Add broccoli and cauliflower. Simmer for 20 minutes, stirring occasionally. Add the champagne, basil, and oregano. Cover and cook for 5 minutes longer.

Place the vegetables and some of the liquid in a blender or food processor, and liquify. Return the mixture to the pan and reheat. Serve hot.

CROQUETTES CAMPO

10-ounce package silken, firm tofu
3 tablespoons flour
Dash of pepper
1 slightly beaten egg
¾ cup bread crumbs, seasoned with parmasan cheese
2 tablespoons olive oil
2 tablespoons Worcestershire sauce
¼ cup unsalted tomato paste
Lemon wedges

Slice tofu into croquette size sections. Arrange slices between two pieces of a thick paper towel to remove moisture. Mix flour and pepper. Dust tofu slices in flour mixture and drop into beaten egg. Sprinkle with bread crumbs. Heat oil in a large, shallow skillet and saute tofu wedges for 2 minutes on each side until a crispy golden texture. Blend Worcestershire sauce and tomato paste. Pour mixture over tofu and serve with small lemon wedges.

EGG SALAD EL GRANADA

2 eggs
1 cup rice
9-ounce can artichoke hearts in water
1 onion
2 cloves garlic
1 large tomato
½ teaspoon dry mustard
½ teaspoon basil
4 tablespoons olive oil
4 tablespoons lemon juice

Hard boil the eggs, cool, peel, and dice.

Prepare the rice according to directions. Let cool to room temperature. Chop the onion and garlic, and cut the tomato into small pieces. Drain artichoke hearts.

Combine these ingredients, and sprinkle with the mustard and basil. Toss briefly with the oil and lemon juice. Serve at room temperature.

EGGS EXETER

1 tablespoon unsalted margarine
4 tablespoons low-fat cottage cheese
4 green onions, minced
1 clove garlic, pressed
4 eggs
Pepper

Melt margarine in skillet. Add cottage cheese. Add onions and garlic. Saute over low flame until browned. Increase heat to medium. Add beaten eggs and scramble until firm. Sprinkle pepper over top, and serve.

Note: For a higher calcium variation, see Eggs Elsinore.

EGGS ELSINORE

1 tablespoon unsalted margarine
15 ounces tofu
4 tablespoons low-fat cottage cheese
4 green onions, minced
1 clove garlic, pressed
4 eggs
Pepper

Melt margarine in skillet. Add tofu and cottage cheese, and mash together. Add onions and garlic. Saute over low flame until browned. Increase heat to medium. Add beaten eggs and scramble until firm. Sprinkle pepper over top and serve.

FETTUCINE SUNLAND

½ pound fettucine
½ cup tofu
1 cup part skim ricotta
⅓ cup onion, chopped
2 cloves garlic, pressed
1 teaspoon Worcestershire sauce
⅛ teaspoon pepper

Preheat oven to 350 F. Cook the pasta following package directions. Drain and mix with remaining ingredients. Pour into a greased 1½-quart casserole. Bake uncovered for 30 minutes, or until a crust forms on top.

FETTUCINE SAUSALITO

1 pound tomatoes
3 tablespoons olive oil
2 cloves garlic
1 tablespoon basil
1 pound fettuccine
1 tablespoon parmesan cheese

Skin tomatoes and cut each one into 6 pieces. Discard seeds. Heat 1 tablespoon olive oil. Add garlic and basil. Saute for 1 minute. Add tomatoes. Cook for 3 minutes more.

Prepare fettuccine as directed on package. Drain thoroughly. Warm 2 tablespoons of olive oil in a large skillet. Place pasta in skillet along with sauce. Cook over medium heat for 3 minutes, stirring occasionally. Transfer to a warm platter, sprinkle with parmesan cheese, and serve at once.

Note: For a higher calcium variation, see Fettucine Felicita Park.

FETTUCINE FELICITA PARK

1 pound tomatoes
3 tablespoons olive oil
2 cloves garlic
1 tablespoon basil
1 pound fettuccine
10 tablespoons romano cheese

Skin tomatoes and cut each one into six pieces. Discard seeds. Heat 1 tablespoon oil. Add garlic and basil. Saute for 1 minute. Add tomatoes. Cook for 3 minutes more.

Prepare fettuccine as directed on package. Drain thoroughly. Warm 2 tablespoons of oil in a large skillet. Place pasta in skillet along with sauce. Cook over medium heat for 3 minutes, stirring occasionally. Transfer to a warm platter, sprinkle with romano cheese, and serve at once.

FRESH FRUIT FRESNO

4 fresh peaches, peeled and pitted
6 fresh apricots, peeled and pitted
8 cherries, pitted
8 slices fresh pineapple
2 bananas
3 tablespoons fructose
8 graham crackers
12 teaspoons triple sec (orange) liqueur
Mint leaves

Cut fruit into bite-size pieces, then sprinkle with fructose. Crush the graham crackers and place at bottom of serving dishes. Spoon fruit on top. Add triple sec. Refrigerate for 1½ hours until set. Serve cold, topped with mint leaves.

FRESH FRUIT SORBET STOVEPIPE WELLS

2 quarts fruit, hulled or pitted
Juice of 1 lemon
1 cup water
1 cup fructose

Place fruit in blender or food processor with half the lemon juice, and puree. Boil the water, then add the fructose, cooking for 5 minutes. Stir in the puree and the rest of the lemon juice.
    Cool, then place in plastic container and freeze.

FRUIT PARFAIT PALA

2 tablespoons honey
Juice of ½ lemon
8 ounces part skim ricotta
4 ounces tofu, cubed
3 cups fresh cherries and pineapple chunks

Mix honey, lemon, and ricotta. In a large bowl, alternate layers of the ricotta mixture with the tofu and fruit. Make four layers. Chill well before serving.

FRUIT SALAD DRESSING SOLEDAD

    1 cup plain low-fat yogurt
    1 cup clover honey
    2 tablespoons grated onion
    2 tablespoons celery seed
    1 tablespoon dry mustard
    1 teaspoon paprika
    1 tablespoon lemon juice

Combine all ingredients. Refrigerate for 1 to 2 hours. Use as a dressing for fresh fruit salad.
    Yield: 2½ cups

FRUIT SORBET RANCHO SANTA FE

    16-ounce container frozen fruit, thawed and pureed
    ¼ cup honey, clover or orange
    1 cup warm water
    1 tablespoon lemon juice

Stirring constantly, combine honey and warm water. Add lemon juice and fruit puree. Freeze till firm.

GAZPACHO GONZALES

    4 firm tomatoes, unpeeled
    2 cloves garlic
    3 tablespoons wine vinegar
    2 tablespoons chives, chopped fine
    2 tablespoons olive oil
    1 small cucumber
    4 tablespoons tomato puree
    1 green chili pepper, chopped fine
    Dash of pepper

Puree all ingredients in a blender or food processor and serve chilled.

GOURMET CHEESE DRESSING GRINGO

8 ounces part-skim ricotta
6 ounces gorgonzola or blue cheese
2 tablespoons safflower oil
1 clove garlic
2 tablespoons lemon juice
1 tablespoon milk

Combine ricotta and gorgonzola or blue cheese. Add oil, garlic, and lemon juice. Beat until well blended. Chill. Add milk. Refrigerate before serving.

Yield: 1½ cups

HALIBUT STEAK WITH CAPERS CAPISTRANO

1 pound halibut steaks, 1-inch thick
Juice of 1 lemon
1 teaspoon margarine
4 tablespoons capers

Rinse the fish under running water and pat dry with a paper towel.

Sprinkle the lemon juice, margarine, and capers on the fish. Broil at 6 inches below the flame, 5 minutes on each side. Serve immediately.

LA JOLLA SHAKE

10-ounce carton soft tofu
2 cups skim milk
½ cup fresh fruit
2 tablespoons fructose
1 tablespoon vanilla extract
5 ice cubes

Place all ingredients in a blender and process until smooth and frothy.

Tofu comes in several types, and we have found that soft tofu is best for the La Jolla Shake. We make ours with Mori-Nu Silken/Soft Tofu and find it makes a delicious shake. If you cannot locate this brand, your grocer may be able to order it for you from Morinaga Nutritional Foods in Los Angeles, California. If you substitute another brand, use only soft tofu.

LASAGNA CHIAMPINO

    2 tablespoons   olive oil
    2 cloves garlic, minced fine
    2 medium sized onions, diced
    6 medium sized tomatoes, skinned and cut in chunks
    1 bay leaf
    ½ cup water
    1 pound lasagna noodles
    ½ pound part-skim mozzarella cheese, sliced
    1 cup part-skim ricotta cheese
    6 tablespoons parmesan cheese
    Dash of pepper

Grease an 8″ × 8″ baking dish with the oil.

Combine garlic, onion, tomato, and bay leaf in a large covered saucepan. Simmer over very low heat for 1½ hours. Add 1½ cups of water when sauce begins to thicken. Stir occasionally. Remove bay leaf.

Preheat oven to 350 F. Prepare lasagna noodles as directed on package, then drain thoroughly. Cover the bottom of the baking dish with one third of the lasagna noodles.

Top with ½ of the mozzarella cheese. Sprinkle with parmesan cheese and dash of pepper. Top with ½ cup of ricotta. Repeat layering process and top with final layer of noodles. Spread the sauce over the top and sprinkle with parmesan cheese. Bake for 50 minutes. Let stand for 10 minutes, so lasagna can set in layers. Cut into 2-inch squares and serve.

LASAGNA LITTLE ITALY

6 ounces tofu
6 ounces part-skim ricotta
1 teaspoon sweet basil
1 pound lasagna noodles
14-ounce can low-sodium tomato sauce
½ pound provolone cheese, sliced thin
¼ pound part-skim mozzarella, sliced
¼ pound mushroom caps, sliced

Preheat oven to 350 F. Combine the tofu and ricotta. Sprinkle with the basil.

Prepare the lasagna noodles according to package directions and drain strips thoroughly. Coat a baking pan with nonstick spray, and spread one third of the tomato sauce on the bottom. Add one third of the pasta and cover with some sauce and one third of the cheeses and mushrooms. Repeat twice, making three layers in all. Bake 45 minutes. Let stand for 10 minutes. Cut into 2-inch squares and serve.

LASAGNA LIVE OAK

6 ounces tofu
6 ounces part-skim ricotta
1 teaspoon basil
1 pound lasagna noodles
14-ounce can low-sodium tomato sauce
6 ounces provolone cheese, sliced thin
¼ pound mushroom caps, sliced

Preheat oven to 350 F. Combine the tofu and ricotta. Sprinkle with the basil.

Prepare the lasagna noodles according to package directions and drain strips thoroughly. Coat a baking pan with nonstick spray, and spread one third of the tomato sauce on the bottom. Add one third of the pasta and cover with some sauce and one third of the cheese mushrooms. Repeat twice, making three layers in all. Bake 45 minutes. Let stand for 10 minutes. Cut into 2-inch squares.

Note: For a higher calcium version of this recipe, see Lasagna Little Italy.

LINGUINE AND CAULIFLOWER CALIFORNIO

    1 pound linguine (made with enriched flour)
    2 tablespoons olive oil
    3 cups cauliflower flowerets
    3 garlic cloves, crushed
    ½ cup part-skim ricotta, at room temperature
    1 ounce provolone cheese, finely diced

Prepare the linguine according to package directions and drain thoroughly. Heat the oil in a large skillet. Add the cauliflower and garlic. Saute for 4 minutes. Cover skillet and heat through for 3 more minutes. Drain the pasta and add it to the skillet. Add the ricotta and provolone and mix well.

LINGUINE CASA LOMA

    1 pound linguine
    4 tablespoons virgin olive oil
    4 cups broccoli flowerets, chopped into small pieces
    4 cloves garlic, crushed
    1½ cups part-skim ricotta
    2 tablespoons basil

Prepare pasta as directed on package and drain thoroughly. While pasta is cooking, heat 2 tablespoons of oil in a skillet. Saute the broccoli and garlic for 4 minutes. Cover and heat 4 minutes more. Stir in the ricotta and basil. Remove from heat. Place pasta in a large serving dish and sprinkle with 2 tablespoons of olive oil and basil. Mix, to prevent sticking. Pour contents of skillet on top of linguine. Toss gently several times. Serve.

   Note: For lower calorie version of this recipe, see Linguine Lafayette.

LINGUINE LAFAYETTE

    ½ pound linguine
    1 tablespoon virgin olive oil
    4 cups broccoli flowerets, chopped into small sections

4 cloves garlic, crushed
1½ cups part-skim ricotta
2 tablespoons basil

Prepare pasta as directed on package and drain thoroughly. While pasta is cooking, heat ½ tablespoon of oil in a skillet. Saute the broccoli and garlic for 4 minutes. Cover and heat 4 minutes more. Stir in the ricotta and basil. Set on side of stove. Place pasta in a large serving dish. Sprinkle with ½ tablespoon of olive oil and the basil. Mix, to prevent sticking. Pour contents of skillet on top of linguine. Toss gently several times. Serve.

MAYONNAISE MALIBU

½ cup tofu
3 tablespoons low-fat yogurt
1 medium egg, boiled
2 teaspoons lemon juice
1 tablespoon green onion, minced
Dash Worcestershire sauce

Mix all ingredients in a blender and let stand 1 hour in refrigerator.

Yield: approximately 1 cup

MUSHROOMS AND PASTA MILL VALLEY

1 pound pasta (any shape)
4 tablespoons olive oil
1 pound mushrooms, sliced
4 cloves garlic, minced
½ pound pearl onions, whole
Pinch of thyme
Pinch of rosemary
Half a lemon

Cook the pasta according to package directions. Drain thoroughly.

Heat the oil and saute the mushrooms, garlic, onions, thyme and rosemary until tender, but not mushy. Toss with the drained pasta. Squeeze the lemon over the mixture, and toss again briefly.

OMELET OJAI

¼ cup nonfat milk
4 eggs, slightly beaten
4 slices monterey jack cheese, shredded
4 ounces tofu, diced
2 tablespoons chives, chopped

Combine the eggs and milk, and pour into a nonstick skillet. When partially set, cover with the cheese and tofu. Fold in half, remove to a serving dish, and sprinkle with chives.

OMELET OCOTILLO

4 ounces tofu, diced
4 eggs, slightly beaten
¼ cup nonfat milk
3½ ounces brie, cubed
1 tablespoon chives, chopped

Combine the eggs and milk, and pour into a nonstick skillet. When partially set, cover with the cheese and tofu. Fold in half, remove to a serving dish, sprinkle with chives, and serve.

Note: For a higher calcium version of this recipe, see Omelet Ojai.

ORANGE ROUGHY OAKLAND

4 fresh Orange Roughy fillets
1 tablespoon olive oil
4 teaspoons capers
1 lemon

Heat broiler for 2 minutes. Drain fish fillets under fresh cold water and dry with paper towel. Place on foil for broiling. Sprinkle with oil and capers. Squeeze whole fresh lemon on top of fish. Pieces of pulp may be added for tartness. Broil for 2 minutes; turn and broil for additional 2 minutes. Serve immediately.

OYSTER COD OCEAN BEACH

    4 tablespoons safflower oil
    6 small white sweet onions, chopped fine
    ½ teaspoon green chili powder
    8-ounce jar of oysters
    ¾ cup fresh Italian bread crumbs
    1½ pounds cod
    Dash of pepper
    Dash of tarragon
    Dash of dill

Preheat oven to 400 F. Heat oil in skillet. Add onion and chili and cook until soft. Dip oysters in crumbs, add to pan, and cook for 5 minutes. Place fish on a greased or nonstick baking pan and spread the oyster mixture over the fish. Sprinkle with pepper, tarragon, and dill. Bake for about 30 minutes.

OYSTER SANDWICH ORLEANS

    8-ounce baguette French bread
    2 8-ounce jars oysters
    3 tablespoons corn meal
    2 tablespoons olive oil
    4 teaspoons mayonnaise
    20–40 drops hot pepper sauce
    ½ lemon

Warm the baguette in the oven, cutting it in half if necessary to fit. Lightly dredge the oysters with the corn meal, and allow them to dry briefly on a rack. Heat the olive oil in a heavy skillet, adding up to 40 drops of hot pepper sauce to it, if desired. Cook the oysters briefly in the oil, no more than 2 minutes per side.

Slice the baguette in half horizontally. Spread the mayonnaise on the insides of both halves. Sprinkle hot pepper sauce on both halves. Place the oysters evenly along the bottom half. Squeeze the lemon juice over them, and then cover them with the top half of the bread. Cut the loaf into serving pieces, and eat.

OYSTERS OCEANSIDE

8-ounce loaf French bread
8 ounces low-fat yogurt
6 tablespoons low-fat milk
¼ cup onion, chopped
1 clove garlic, minced
¼ teaspoon Worcestershire sauce
8-ounce can smoked oysters

Slice the bread and brown it in a 350 F. oven for 10 minutes until crisp. Place the slices on a baking dish.

Blend the yogurt and milk, and fold in the remaining ingredients. Spoon onto the bread slices. Broil for about 3 minutes, or until slightly browned.

OYSTERS PIRATE'S COVE

8-ounce loaf French bread
4 ounces plain low-fat yogurt
6 ounces water and oyster juice
¼ cup onion, chopped
1 clove garlic, minced
¼ teaspoon Worcestershire sauce
8-ounce can smoked oysters

Slice the bread and brown it in a 350 F. oven for 10 minutes, until crisp. Place the slices on a baking dish.

Thin the yogurt with the water and oyster juice, and fold in the remaining ingredients. Spoon onto the bread slices. Broil for about 3 minutes, or until slightly browned.

Note: For a higher calcium version of this recipe, see Oysters Oceanside.

PASTA AND CHEESE CUCAMONGA

⅓ cup onion, minced
2 tablespoons safflower margarine
1 cup soft bread crumbs
1 cup Sauce Rancho Mirage (see page 196)
2 cups pasta (any shape)
4 ounces part skim mozzarella cheese or Bel Paese

Preheat oven to 350 F. Grease a 2-quart casserole.

Saute onion in margarine in a skillet. Add ½ cup of the bread crumbs and stir until brown. Set crumb mixture aside. Add Sauce Rancho Mirage to mixture.

Boil pasta as intructed on package and drain thoroughly. Place half of it in the greased casserole and cover with half of the crumb mixture. Repeat with the rest of the pasta and crumbs. Cover top with cheese and the remainder of the bread crumbs. Bake for 20 minutes, or until cheese is melted and crumbs are lightly browned.

PASTA BROCCOLI BOLINAS

1 pound linguine
1½ pounds broccoli
4 quarts water
¼ cup olive oil
3 cloves garlic
Generous dash of pepper
4 tablespoons romano cheese

Cook linguine as directed on package. Drain thoroughly, saving three cups of the liquid.

Prepare broccoli tops, leaving only enough of the stems to secure bouquets. Steam briefly, about 2 minutes. When finished, lay aside.

Heat olive oil in large saucepan. Saute garlic until soft. Add broccoli and liquid. Season with pepper. Simmer over low heat for 10 minutes. Serve over linguine. Sprinkle with romano cheese.

PASTA FIESTA ISLAND

6 ounces pasta (any shape)
4 ounces frozen corn kernels
7 ounces cooked ham, diced
4-ounce can diced green chiles
7 ounces green chile salsa
1 large tomato

Cook the pasta and the corn according to package directions. Drain each and allow to cool.

Combine the ham, pasta, and corn in a large serving bowl. Mix in the chiles and the salsa. Slice the tomato into wedges and arrange over the top of the mixture. Serve at room temperature.

PASTA GARDEN VEGETABLE SAN FERNANDO

2 cups sliced baby carrots
8 baby turnips
16 ounces cooked tiny pasta shells
1 cup plain low-fat yogurt

Microwave the carrots and turnips for about 1 minute in a covered dish, or steam over water until tender firm. Cool.

Mix with pasta and yogurt, and chill.

PASTA MADERA

1 cup mushrooms, sliced
8 ounces rotelli, cooked (spiral pasta)
¼ cup pimiento, finely cut
8 ounces cheddar cheese, cubed
1 cup nonfat milk
3 tablespoons onion, chopped
Mustard to taste
1 teaspoon Worcestershire sauce
1 teaspoon pepper
1 tomato, sliced

Steam the mushrooms and onions in a covered saucepan until soft. Mix with the rotelli and pimiento and place in a nonstick 1½-quart casserole.

Heat the cheese, milk, mustard, Worcestershire sauce, and pepper in a saucepan until the cheese melts. (This can be done in a microwave.) Stir half of the mixture into the pasta, and top with the tomato. Pour the rest of the mixture on top. Bake for 25 minutes, or until bubbly hot.

PASTA NUEVO

> 1 pound egg noodles
> 2 tablespoons safflower margarine, melted
> 4 cups cabbage, sliced in thin sections
> ½ cup water
> 1 cup scallions, chopped fine

Cook noodles as directed on package. Drain. Warm oil in large skillet. Saute cabbage 3–4 minutes. Add water. Cover and simmer for 4 minutes. Place noodles on top of cabbage. Steam for 5 minutes.

Mix cabbage and noodles together and top with scallions. Serve at once.

PASTA PENASQUITOS

> 1 cup mushrooms, sliced
> 8 ounces rotelli, cooked (spiral pasta)
> ¼ cup pimiento, finely cut
> 4 ounces cheddar cheese, cubed
> 1 cup nonfat milk
> 3 tablespoons garlic, chopped
> 1 teaspoon pepper
> 1 tomato, sliced

Steam the mushrooms and garlic in a covered saucepan until soft. Mix with the rotelli and place in a nonstick 1½-quart casserole.

Heat the cheese, milk, and pepper in a saucepan until the cheese melts. (This can be done in a microwave.) Stir half of the mixture into the pasta, and top with the tomato. Pour the rest of the mixture on top. Bake for 25 minutes, or until bubbly hot.

Note: For a higher calcium variation, see Pasta Madera.

PASTA SHELLS SICILIANO

½ pound jumbo pasta shells
32-ounce can low-sodium tomato puree
1 teaspoon basil
1 teaspoon oregano
2 10-ounce packages silken/soft tofu
4 ounces part skim mozzarella cheese, shredded
¼ cup parmesan cheese, grated

Preheat the oven to 350 F. Cook the pasta according to directions on the package. Drain.

Mix the tomato puree with the basil and oregano. Line a 13 × 9 × 2inch baking dish with half of the tomato sauce. Mix the tofu, mozzarella and parmesan. Place the cooked shells side by side in the pan in a single layer, and spoon the mixture into them. Pour the remaining sauce over the shells. Bake for 30 minutes or until the shells are thoroughly heated.

PEACHES PACIFICA

8 graham crackers, crushed
3 tablespoons safflower margarine, melted
6 large ripe peaches, pitted and cut in half
12 tablespoons Marsala wine or sherry
2 tablespoons lemon juice
2 tablespoons water
4 tablespoons fructose

Preheat oven to 375 F. Turn over the crushed graham crackers in the melted margarine, then line a shallow baking dish with the mixture. Place the peaches in the dish, cut side down. Combine the wine and lemon juice, pouring some over each half. Bake for a total of 30 minutes. After the first 15 minutes, pour the water over the peaches, to prevent scorching.

Five minutes before removing the dish from the oven, sprinkle the peaches with fructose. Serve warm.

PEACHES PARADISE VALLEY

    4 large fresh peaches, peeled and cut into small chunks
    ½ cup orange honey
    2 tablespoons lemon juice
    Pinch of ginger

In serving dish combine all ingredients and let flavors blend for at least ½ hour. Serve at room temperature.

PEARS PEARLDALE

    6 fresh pears
    ½ cup red California wine
    1 teaspoon cinnamon
    ¼ cup clover honey
    1 tablespoon lemon juice
    Fresh mint sprigs

Peel and core the pears. Cut into lengthwise halves. In a double boiler, stir wine, cinnamon, honey, and lemon juice for 1 minute. Gently add the pear halves, two at a time, and cook in sauce briefly, just until tender. Chill and serve topped with fresh mint.

PIZZA PALOMAR

    1 pound fresh mushrooms
    6 tablespoons olive oil
    6 fresh tomatoes, skinned and cut into one inch
    sections
    2 cloves of garlic, finely chopped
    2 tablespoons oregano
    2 tablespoons basil
    2 tablespoons capers
    Dash of fresh black pepper
    2 tablespoons parsley, chopped
    8 English muffins

Trim the bottoms of the mushroom stems, then slice the mushrooms in half, lengthwise.

Saute tomatoes in 4 tablespoons oil with garlic, oregano, sweet basil, capers, pepper, and parsley for 15 minutes. Add mushrooms. Simmer 20 minutes more over low flame.

Preheat broiler. Cut muffins in half and place on baking sheets, cut sides up. Top with tomato mixture.

Broil until warm and tomato sauce bubbles.

POPPYSEED DRESSING CALIFORNIA

1 cup orange honey
1 teaspoon dry mustard
⅔ cup vinegar
3 tablespoons onion juice
2 tablespoons safflower oil
2 tablespoons lemon juice
3 tablespoons poppyseeds
2 tablespoons water, if necessary

Mix honey, mustard, and vinegar. Stir in onion juice. Slowly add oil, beating constantly until thick. (You may also prepare in blender or food processor.) Stir in poppyseeds. Thin with water, if necessary.

Yield: 2¼ cups

RAVIOLI RIVERSIDE

2 cups bread crumbs, made from slightly stale French bread
1 pound frozen ricotta-filled ravioli (available at specialty stores)
2 cups nonfat milk
5 tablespoons parmesan cheese
2 tablespoons safflower oil

Preheat oven to 350 F. Sprinkle thin layer of bread crumbs evenly in bottom of deep pan. Dip ravioli into milk and place close together on top of breading. Repeat layers until pan is full. Sprinkle with parmesan cheese. Pour safflower oil on top. Bake until golden brown, about 20 minutes.

RED CABBAGE RESEDA

1 red cabbage, cored and chopped
2 large apples, peeled, cored, and diced
1 tablespoon caraway seed
1 teaspoon malt vinegar
⅛ teaspoon pepper

Mix all ingredients. Simmer over low heat, stirring occasionally, for about 25 minutes.

RED SNAPPER WITH VEGETABLES VISTA

½ pound turnips
½ pound cucumber, peeled
½ pound mushrooms
1 pound broccoli
1 teaspoon cumin
2 teaspoons oregano
4 fillets red snapper (about 1 pound)
1 lime
4 sprigs fresh cilantro

Cut the turnips and cucumber into small cubes and place in a casserole. Rinse the mushrooms, slice, and add. Trim the broccoli, separate into flowerets, and add. Sprinkle with cumin and oregano, and cover.

Rinse the fish under running water and pat dry with a paper towel. Half-fill a large skillet with water and squeeze one fourth of the lime into it. Cut the remainder of the lime into four wedges. Measure the thickness of the fish. Place a large nonstick trivet in the skillet water, and place the fish fillets on it. Cover the fillets with the cilantro sprigs, and cover the pan. Bring the water to a boil, then turn down the heat and steam the fish for 10 minutes per inch of fish thickness.

Cook the vegetables in a microwave on high for about 4 minutes, or until tender firm, or until you can smell the spices.

Apportion the vegetables on warmed plates, and place the fish on top. Garnish with lime wedges.

RICE PILAF RANCHITA

½ cup long grain white rice
1 cup unsalted chicken broth (preferably homemade)
½ teaspoon thyme
½ teaspoon marjoram

Combine all ingredients, cover, and bring to a boil. Simmer 17 minutes. Let stand 10 minutes covered. Serve.

SALMON SANTA CRUZ

1 pound canned Pacific salmon
1 egg, beaten
1 large onion, chopped
Juice of 1 lemon
1½ cups part-skim ricotta
Marjoram
Thyme
Pepper
4 slices provolone cheese

Preheat oven to 350 F. Blend the salmon in a bowl with the egg. Add the onion and the juice of the lemon. Mix in the ricotta, herbs, and pepper. Transfer mixture to a loaf pan and top with the cheese. Bake for 40 minutes, covered. Remove cover and bake 10 minutes longer.

SALMON SAUSALITO

1 pound Pacific salmon steaks, 1-inch thick
Juice of half a lemon
1 teaspoon olive oil
1 teaspoon oregano
1 teaspoon thyme
1 teaspoon basil
1 teaspoon rosemary

Rinse the fish under running water and pat dry with a paper towel. Sprinkle with lemon juice, olive oil, and herbs, and broil the fish 6 inches below the flame for 5 minutes on each side. Serve immediately.

SALMON SEACLIFF

    1 pound canned Pacific salmon
    1 egg, beaten
    1 large onion, chopped
    Juice of 1 lemon
    ¾ cup part-skim ricotta
    Marjoram
    Thyme
    Pepper
    2 slices provolone cheese

Preheat oven to 350 F. Blend the salmon in a bowl with the egg. Add the onion and the juice of the lemon. Mix in the ricotta, herbs, and pepper. Transfer mixture to a loaf pan and top with the cheese. Bake for 40 minutes, covered. Remove cover and bake 10 minutes longer.

    Note: For a higher calcium version of this recipe, see Salmon Santa Cruz.

SALMON SHELL BEACH

    1 pound Pacific canned salmon
    1 cup nonfat milk
    1 egg beaten
    3 tablespoons shallots, minced
    2 teaspoons poultry seasoning
    ½ teaspoon tarragon
    Corn oil margarine
    Lemon wedges

Preheat oven to 375 F. Mix salmon and milk in a bowl. Add egg and remaining ingredients and mix well. Transfer the mixture to a loaf pan greased with corn oil margarine. Bake for about 40 minutes.

    Serve this aromatic seafood loaf with lemon wedges surrounding it. The delicate meat will give no hint that it has not come straight from the ocean to your kitchen.

SALMON MOLD SAN CARLOS

    16-ounce can pink Pacific salmon
    ½ cup cucumber, seeded and diced
    ¼ cup onion, chopped fine
    2 envelopes unflavored gelatin
    ½ cup cold water
    ½ cup tomato paste
    ¼ cup apple vinegar
    1 cup plus 2 tablespoons plain low-fat yogurt

Drain salmon, saving the liquid. Flake and mix the salmon with cucumber and onion. Soften gelatin in cold water. Combine salmon liquid, tomato paste, and vinegar in a saucepan, and bring to a boil. Stir in the softened gelatin until dissolved. Blend this into the salmon mixture. Stir in 1 cup of yogurt.

Coat the inside of a 1-quart fish mold with 2 tablespoons yogurt, and fill with salmon mixture. Chill until firm. Unmold onto serving platter.

SAUCE RANCHO MIRAGE

    2 cloves garlic, minced
    4 tablespoons olive oil
    2 cups part-skim ricotta
    Juice of 1 large lemon squeezed
    2 teaspoons dry mustard
    2 teaspoons wine vinegar
    1 tablespoon mayonnaise
    Dash of pepper

Saute garlic in 2 tablespoons oil. Heat ricotta in double boiler. Add warm garlic and olive oil mixture and all other ingredients to the ricotta. Cook in double boiler for 15 minutes over medium-low flame, stirring occasionally. Serve at once over warm vegetables.

Note: Perfect for asparagus and broccoli. Adds a zesty flair to any vegetable. Also use as a replacement for white sauce.

SCALLOPS SAN SIMEON

1 teaspoon margarine
¾ pounds scallops
½ cup soft bread crumbs
⅛ teaspoon pepper
1 tablespoon anise
½ cup plain low-fat yogurt

Coat the bottom of a square baking pan with the margarine. Wash the scallops, drain, and dry on paper towels. Cut the scallops in half if they are very large. Place half the scallops in the pan and cover with half of the bread crumbs, pepper, and anise. Repeat. Pour the yogurt over the top and bake for 30 minutes at 350 F.

SEAFOOD STRATA SANTA MONICA

10-ounce package frozen shrimp, thawed
4 cups nonfat milk
3 eggs
4 tablespoons California sherry
1 tablespoon dry mustard
8 ounces fresh crab meat
Margarine
6 slices slightly stale Italian bread
2 cups parmesan cheese, grated

Quarter each slice of bread and dab with margarine. Mix shrimp, milk, eggs, sherry, mustard, and crab meat. Grease casserole with margarine. Alternate layers of bread, cheese, and shrimp mixture. Chill overnight or for a few hours. Bake at 350 F. for 1 hour.

SEAFOOD STRATA SUNSET BEACH

10-ounce package frozen shrimp, thawed
4 cups nonfat milk
1 egg
4 tablespoons California sherry
1 tablespoon dry mustard
8 ounces fresh crab meat
Margarine
6 slices slightly stale Italian bread

Quarter each slice of bread and dab with margarine. Mix shrimp, milk, egg, sherry, mustard, and crab meat. Grease casserole with margarine. Alternate layers of bread with shrimp mixture. Chill overnight or for a few hours. Bake at 350 F. for 1 hour.

Note: For a higher calcium version of this recipe, see Seafood Strata Santa Monica.

SEA SALAD SEAL BEACH

> 14 ounces small, cooked shrimp
> 7 ounces crab meat, chopped
> 1½ cups cucumber, chopped and seeded
> ½ teaspoon pepper
> 2 tablespoons onion, chopped
> 1½ teaspoons Worcestershire sauce
> Lettuce salad or 4 large tomatoes

Mix shrimp, crab meat, cucumber, pepper, onion and Worchestershire sauce. Chill. Serve on lettuce or use to stuff tomatoes.

SHAD SHELTER COVE

> 2 teaspoons safflower margarine
> 1½ pounds shad, boned
> Juice of 1 lemon
> Dash of pepper
> Dash of anise
> 2 cups plain low-fat yogurt

Preheat oven to 400 F. Grease baking dish with margarine. Put shad in dish and sprinkle it with lemon juice, pepper, and anise. Bake uncovered for 15–20 minutes. Fold yogurt over fish, then bake for another 10 minutes.

SHRIMP DIP DIAMOND SPRINGS

> 2 tablespoons safflower oil
> 1 tablespoon anchovy paste
> 1 tablespoon green onion, minced
> 2 tablespoons tarragon vinegar
> 1 pound medium shrimp, cooked and chilled

Mix together the safflower oil, anchovy paste, onion, and vinegar. Chill. Serve as a dip with the shrimp.

SHRIMP IN TOMATO BEDS TEHAMA

    4 large, firm tomatoes
    2 tablespoons olive oil
    1 medium-size white onion, minced
    10 ounces cooked or canned shrimp
    2 tablespoons basil
    1 cup cheese-flavored bread crumbs
    Dash of pepper
    4 tablespoons parmesan cheese

Heat oven to 325 F. Slice off the top ends of the tomatoes, core the centers, and turn upside down to permit them to dry. Heat the oil in a skillet, add the onion and saute until onion is shiny. Add the shrimp, basil, crumbs, and pepper. Heat thoroughly. Fill tomatoes with the combination and sprinkle with cheese. Bake 15 minutes. Serve heated or chilled.

SHRIMP LAGUNA BEACH

    1 pound shrimp
    Dill weed
    4 slices French bread
    1½ tablespoons chives
    Pinch of pepper
    ¼ cup plain low-fat yogurt
    1 tablespoon lemon juice
    1 tablespoon flour

Place the shrimp in cold water with dill weed, bring to a boil, and simmer 10 minutes.

Remove crusts from the bread and make bread crumbs. Mix in the chives.

Preheat the oven to 375 F. Drain the shrimp and let cool. Mix with the pepper, yogurt, lemon juice, and flour, and place in a greased baking dish. Sprinkle the bread crumbs on top. Bake for 20 minutes.

SHRIMP BARBECUE MONTEREY

½ cup soy sauce
¼ cup olive oil
½ cup sherry
2 tablespoons lemon juice
1 teaspoon basil
1 teaspoon oregano
2 pounds shrimp

Mix all ingredients except shrimp. Pour marinade over shrimp. Refrigerate for 3–4 hours. Thread shrimp on bamboo skewers and grill over coals or place under broiler.

SHRIMP WITH PASTA SAN LUIS REY

8 ounces tiny pasta shells
2 tablespoons scallions, chopped
1 slice lemon
1 bay leaf
4 cups water
1 pound raw shrimp, peeled and deveined
1 tablespoon olive oil
1 tablespoon flour
1 8-ounce can tomato sauce
2 cloves garlic
1 tablespoon margarine

Cook pasta according to package directions. Drain. Place scallions, lemon, bay leaf, and water in a pot. Bring to a boil, add shrimp, and simmer 5 minutes. Drain, reserving the liquid. Heat oil in a saucepan. Stir in reserved liquid and flour, tomato sauce, and garlic. Bring to a boil. Stir in shrimp and leave on flame until completely heated.

Toss pasta with margarine. Serve the shrimp over it.

SOLE MARINA DEL REY

1 pound filet of sole
2 tablespoons olive oil
Juice of 1 lemon
Fresh rosemary
Pepper

Preheat oven to 350 F. Rinse the fish under running water and pat dry with a paper towel. Grease a baking dish with 1 teaspoon of the oil. Combine the lemon juice, rosemary, and pepper with the rest of the oil and marinate the fish in it for 2–4 hours. Remove from the marinade and place the fish in the baking dish. Bake for 35 minutes. If desired, garnish with additional fresh rosemary.

SPAGHETTI SAN FRANCISCO

1 pound tomatoes
1 pound fresh mushrooms
1 tablespoon olive oil
1–2 cloves garlic, diced
Pepper to taste
1–2 teaspoon oregano
1–2 teaspoon basil
8 ounces enriched spaghetti
½ cup grated parmesan cheese

Puree the tomatoes in a food processor or blender or cut in a fine dice. Steam mushrooms until tender. Combine these ingredients in a pan, add the olive oil, garlic, pepper, oregano, and basil, and cook covered for 30 mintes over low heat. Thin with water, if needed.

Cook the spaghetti and drain. Place on a serving dish and pour the sauce over it. Top with cheese.

SPAGHETTI SANTA NELLA

2 pounds tomatoes
1 pound fresh mushrooms
1 tablespoon olive oil
1–2 cloves garlic, diced
Pepper to taste
2–4 teaspoons oregano
2–4 teaspoons basil
1 pound enriched spaghetti
½ cup grated parmesan cheese

Puree the tomatoes in a food processor or blender, or cut in a fine dice. Steam mushrooms until tender. Combine these ingredients in a pan, add the oil, garlic, pepper, oregano, and basil, and cook covered for 30 minutes over low heat. Thin with water, if needed.

Cook the spaghetti and drain. Place on a serving dish and pour the sauce over it. Top with cheese.

Note: For a lower calorie version of this recipe, see Spaghetti San Francisco.

SPAGHETTINI WITH CLAM SAUCE PISMO BEACH

¼ cup olive oil
2 cloves of garlic, minced
½ tablespoon oregano
Dash of pepper
1 cup little neck clams, with juice
½ cup water
1 pound spaghettini (thin spaghetti)

Heat oil in saucepan and saute garlic, oregano, and pepper. Add the clams with their water and cook until clams are tender, about 30 minutes. Add water, if necessary.

Prepare spaghettini as directed on package and drain thoroughly. Place spaghettini on warm platter and spoon clam sauce over it.

Note: For a higher calcium version of this recipe, see Spaghettini with Clam Sauce Sonoma.

SPAGHETTINI WITH CLAM SAUCE SONOMA

¼ cup olive oil
2 cloves garlic, minced
½ tablespoon oregano
Dash of pepper
1 cup little neck clams, with juice
½ cup water
1 pound spaghettini (thin spaghetti)
½ cup parmesan cheese

Heat oil in saucepan and saute garlic, oregano, and pepper. Add the clams with their water and cook until clams are tender, about 30 minutes. Add water, if necessary.

Prepare spaghettini as directed on package and drain thoroughly. Place spaghettini on warm platter and spoon clam sauce over it. Sprinkle with parmesan cheese.

STRAWBERRY-CHAMPAGNE MOLD
STRAWBERRY CREEK

1 quart strawberries
½ cup fructose
½ cup California champagne
2 envelopes unflavored gelatin
½ cup cold water
½ cup water, boiled
2 egg whites

Reserve a few strawberries with stems, for garnish. Hull the remainder of the strawberries and puree in a blender or food processor. Continue processing while adding fructose and champagne. Place the mixture in a bowl and chill in the refrigerator.

Soften the gelatin in cold water, then add the hot water. Chill in the refrigerator till cool but not set.

Combine the gelatin and cold strawberries, beating until slightly thick and fluffy. Whip the egg whites until almost stiff, then fold into the fruit mixture.

Place in a 2-quart mold and refrigerate for 3½ hours. For serving, turn the mold out on a chilled platter and surround it with the reserved whole strawberries.

STUFFED EGGS ESCONDIDO

4 eggs, hard cooked
4 ounces canned, smoked sardines
2 tablespoons lemon juice
Pepper
Paprika
4 sprigs cilantro

Peel the eggs and half lengthwise. Remove the yolks and mash with the sardines, lemon juice, pepper, and paprika. Fill egg whites with the mixture. Garnish with additional paprika or whole leaves of cilantro.

TACOS TEMECULA

6 tomatoes, medium-sized
12 ounces part skim-milk mozzarella, sliced in thin segments
2 onions, medium sized, chopped
1 bouquet of cilantro, chopped
4 tablespoons olive oil
Dash of pepper
8 corn tortillas, medium-sized

Cut tomatoes into 1-inch cubes and saute them with the onions and cilantro in 2 tablespoons oil for 15 minutes. Add pepper.

Lay tortillas on baking sheet. Place tomato mixture and cheese on center of each. Fold into half-moon shapes. Heat the remaining oil in a skillet and fry tortillas on both sides until crisp and brown. Drain on paper towels and serve immediately.

TACOS TRUCKEE

8 corn tortillas, medium-sized
6 tomatoes, medium-sized
2-ounces part-skim mozzarella cheese, sliced in thin segments
2 onions, medium sized, chopped
1 bouquet of cilantro, chopped
4 tablespoons olive oil
Dash of pepper

Cut tomatoes into 1-inch cubes and saute them with the tomatoes, onions, and cilantro in 2 tablespoons oil for 15 minutes.

Lay tortillas on baking sheet. Place tomato mixture and cheese on center of each. Fold into half-moon shapes. Heat the remaining oil in a skillet and fry tortillas on both sides until crisp and brown. Drain on paper towels and serve immediately.

Note: For a higher calcium variation, see Tacos Temecula.

TROUT TWIN BRIDGES

> 1 tablespoon olive oil
> 6 scallions, chopped fine
> 1 tablespoon basil
> 2 bay leaves, crumpled
> ½ cup white wine
> 1 cup water
> 1 pound rainbow trout, in 4 pieces

Heat oil and saute the scallions. Add the bay leaves and basil. When the scallions are soft, add the wine and water, and simmer covered for 5 minutes. Place the trout in the mixture, cover, and cook for 10 minutes. Keep the heat high, but avoid boiling. Remove the fish to plates, and pour some of the sauce over it.

TURNIPS TIBURON

> 12 baby turnips
> 4 tomatoes, cut in wedges
> 4 teaspoons olive oil
> 8 tablespoons part-skim ricotta
> 8 tablespoons chopped chives

Quarter the turnips and microwave covered for 1 minute, or steam 5–10 minutes. Drain if necessary. Add tomato wedges and mix gently with oil. Cool. Mix with ricotta and chives. Chill.

VEGETABLE CAVIAR VIOLA

> 4 small zucchini
> 1 tablespoon olive oil
> 2 small onions, chopped
> 1 tomato, chopped
> ½ pound cauliflower, chopped fine
> ½ pound broccoli flowerets, chopped
> 1 tablespoon lemon juice
> ½ teaspoon oregano
> ½ teaspoon basil
> ¼ teaspoon pepper

Slice the zucchini into rounds, then quarter the pieces. Heat the oil and saute the zucchini with the onions, tomato, cauliflower, broccoli, lemon juice, herbs, and pepper. Mix thoroughly. Let cool slightly before serving.

Note: For a higher calcium version of this recipe, see Vegetable Caviar Ventura.

VEGETABLE CAVIAR VENTURA

4 small zucchini
1 tablespoon olive oil
2 small onions, chopped
1 tomato, chopped
½ pound cauliflower, chopped fine
½ pound broccoli flowerets, chopped
1 tablespoon lemon juice
½ teaspoon oregano
½ teaspoon basil
¼ teaspoon pepper
10 ounces tofu, diced
8 ounces plain low-fat yogurt

Slice the zucchini into rounds, then quarter the pieces. Heat the oil and saute the zucchini with the onions, tomato, cauliflower, broccoli, lemon juice, herbs, and pepper. Mix thoroughly. Let cool slightly, then add the tofu and yogurt.

VEGETABLE LOAVES VENICE

1½ 10-ounce packages tofu, drained
1 clove garlic, chopped
1 tablespoon fresh chives, minced
½ cup bread crumbs, seasoned with oregano and basil
1 beaten egg
Pinch of black pepper
1 tomato, pureed
1 teaspoon oregano
1 teaspoon basil (optional)
2 tablespoons romano cheese, grated

Preheat oven to 350 F. Blend tofu, garlic, chives, seasoned crumbs, egg, and pepper. Mold into 1½-inch diameter balls. Place the balls in a greased, nonstick pan and saute until crisp looking. Transfer them to a loaf pan, pour tomato puree over them and sprinkle with oregano (and basil) and grated cheese. Bake for 15 minutes. Serve hot or cold, or with spaghetti.

VEGETABLE-YOGURT LOAF TAHOE

> 2 cloves garlic, minced
> 2 tablespoons fresh chives, minced
> 10 mushrooms, thinly sliced
> 2 tomatoes, thinly sliced
> 12 ounces plain low-fat yogurt
> 20 ounces tofu, cut in ½-inch cubes
> ½ cup parmesan

Preheat oven to 350 F. Saute garlic and chives in a lightly greased, nonstick pan until tender. Combine with mushrooms and tomatoes in a bowl and mix gently. Place half of the mixture on the bottom of a greased, nonstick loaf pan. Pour half of the yogurt on top and add a layer of half the tofu. Pour one-fourth of the yogurt over the tofu. Layer balance of ingredients in the same sequence. Bake for 30 minutes.

Serve with the parmesan.

VEGETABLE-YOGURT LOAF TECOPA

> 2 cloves garlic, minced
> 2 tablespoons fresh chives, minced
> 10 mushrooms, thinly sliced
> 2 tomatoes, thinly sliced
> 6 ounces low-fat yogurt
> 10 ounces tofu, cut in ½-inch cubes

Preheat oven to 350 F. Saute garlic and chives in a lightly greased, nonstick pan until tender. Combine with mushrooms and tomatoes in a bowl and mix gently. Place half of the mixture on the bottom of a greased, nonstick loaf pan. Pour half of the yogurt on top and add a layer of half the tofu. Pour one-fourth of the yogurt over the tofu. Layer balance of ingredients in the same sequence. Bake for 30 minutes.

Note: For a higher calcium version of this recipe, see Vegetable-Yogurt Loaf Tahoe.

VEGETABLES CHINATOWN

1 pound egg noodles
½ pound snow peas
¾ pound bean sprouts
6-ounce can water chestnuts, drained
1 cup cucumber, chopped fine and seeded
1 cup grated carrots
8-ounce packages tofu
2 tablespoons olive oil
4 small green onions, chopped fine

Cook noodles as directed on the package and drain. Cook all the vegetables in a steamer until almost tender. Dice the tofu into ½-inch cubes. Heat the oil in a skillet and add the vegetables and tofu. Cook over a low flame just until hot.

Place the noodles on a serving dish, cover with the vegetables, and serve immediately.

VERMICELLI WITH SAUCE SAN BRUNO

6 tomatoes, medium-sized
1 pound vermicelli (sometimes called fidelini)
2 cloves of garlic, minced
2 onions, medium-sized, diced
1 tablespoon oregano
1 tablespoon basil
4 tablespoons olive oil

Bring water to a boil and immerse tomatoes for a split second, to make it easy to remove skins. Cut the tomatoes into 1-inch cubes.

Cook vermicelli as instructed on package and drain thoroughly.

Saute the garlic, onion, oregano, and basil in the oil in a large skillet. Add tomatoes and cook over medium heat for 15 minutes, stirring occasionally, but avoid mashing tomatoes.

Serve pasta on a heated platter topped with sauce.

Note: For a higher calcium version of this recipe, see Vermicelli with Sauce Sorrento Valley.

VERMICELLI WITH SAUCE SORRENTO VALLEY

6 tomatoes, medium-sized
1 pound vermicelli (sometimes called fidelini)
2 cloves of garlic, minced
2 onions, medium-sized, diced
1 tablespoon oregano
1 tablespoon basil
4 tablespoons olive oil
8 tablespoons parmesan

Bring water to a boil and immerse tomatoes for a split second, to make it easy to remove skins. Cut the tomatoes into 1-inch cubes.

Cook vermicelli as instructed on package and drain thoroughly.

Saute the garlic, onion, oregano, and basil in the oil in a large skillet. Add tomatoes and cook over medium heat for 15 minutes, stirring occasionally, but avoid mashing tomatoes.

Serve pasta on a heated platter topped with sauce and sprinkled with parmesan cheese.

WHIPPED DELIGHT WHITTIER

15 ounces tofu
3 tablespoons orange honey
2½ teaspoons vanilla extract

Blend all ingredients until smooth. Serve as topping on fruit.

ZUCCHINI-MUSHROOM SALAD SAN JOAQUIN

1 pound zucchini
1 pound mushrooms
2 tablespoons chives
Oregano
Basil
1½ cups croutons
Juice of 1 lemon

Slice the vegetables, and mix with herbs and croutons. Squeeze lemon over them, and let stand for 15 minutes.

Appendix A

A Calcium Counter of Absorbable (Usable) Calcium

The Calcium Counter lists basic foods alphabetically so that you can quickly look up the calcium content of many foods. To figure out the calcium content in a prepared food, such as apple pie, look up the separate ingredients— the amount of apples, sugar, flour, and shortening in a serving— and add the calcium amounts. If you calculate it directly from the table, it will be much more accurate than if we try to measure it for you because recipes and portion sizes vary widely. Don't rely on calcium counters published in other books. All such counters report the *total* calcium in a food or recipe, rather than the usable calcium, or calcium that the body is able to absorb. In a given food, much of the reported calcium may be completely unusable, making your calcium count woefully inaccurate.

Most people tend to eat the same things repeatedly. Once you calculate the calcium content of your favorite prepared foods, write it in a notebook or diary and you won't have to do the calculations again.

By picking high-calcium sources and varying the food groups, you can put together a balanced high-calcium diet of your own. There are some foods for which data on compounds that bind calcium are unavailable; these are marked with an asterisk (*).

Food	True calcium available mg per 100 g	Calories	% fat
Abalone*	37	98	1
Albacore	26	177	8
Almonds, dried	− 33	598	54
Anchovy, pickled	168	176	10
Apple juice, bottled	1	47	0
Apples	7	58	1
Apple sauce*	4	91	0
Apricots	14	86	0
Artichokes	47	26	0
Asparagus	20	20	0
Avocados	10	167	16
Bacon, Canadian	14	277	18
Bacon	14	611	52
Bamboo shoots*	13	27	0
Bananas	8	85	0
Barley	− 90	348	1
Beans, canned, red	16	90	0
Beans, lima*	47	111	1
Beans, mung*	17	28	0
Beans, snap, wax*	50	22	0
Beans, young, green in pod	− 20	25	0
Beef, corned, medium fat	20	216	12
Beef, rump, roasted	10	317	23
Beer, 4.5% alcohol, 8 oz.	− 20	42	0
Beets	− 34	32	0
Biscuits, baking powder	121	369	17
Blackberries	24	58	1
Blueberries	8	62	1
Boysenberries	25	48	0
Bran, wheat	− 350	240	3

Food	True calcium available mg per 100 g	Calories	% fat
Brazil nuts	−198	654	67
Bread, French	43	290	3
Bread, white	68	269	3
Bread, whole-wheat	33	241	3
Broccoli	103	32	0
Brussels sprouts	33	36	0
Brussels sprouts, boiled	31	45	0
Bulgur (parboiled wheat)	−35	182	3
Bullhead, black	0	84	2
Burbot	0	82	1
Butter	20	716	81
Butterfish	0	169	10
Buttermilk	121	36	0
Cabbage, green	49	24	0
Cabbage, red	39	31	0
Cabbage, savoy*	65	24	0
Cantaloupe*	13	30	0
Carp	50	115	4
Carrots, boiled	26	31	0
Carrots, raw	31	42	0
Casaba melon*	14	27	0
Catsup	22	106	0
Cauliflower	20	22	0
Caviar, sturgeon	276	262	15
Celery	34	17	0
Chard, Swiss	−220	25	0
Cheese, American, processed	697	370	30
Cheese, blue or Roquefort	315	368	31
Cheese, brick	730	370	31
Cheese, Brie	185	334	30
Cheese, Camembert	105	299	25
Cheese, cheddar	750	398	32
Cheese, cottage, creamed	94	106	4
Cheese, cottage, uncreamed	90	86	0
Cheese, cream	62	374	38
Cheese, Edam	739	354	26
Cheese, feta	500	262	20
Cheese, fontina	557	385	29
Cheese, goat	405	426	28

Food	True calcium available mg per 100 g	Calories	% fat
Cheese, Gouda	707	354	26
Cheese, Gruyère	1,025	410	30
Cheese, Limburger	590	354	28
Cheese, monterey jack	757	371	29
Cheese, mozzarella	525	280	20
Cheese, mozzarella (low moisture)	582	315	23
Cheese, mozzarella (low moisture, part skim)	739	276	16
Cheese, Muenster	725	364	28
Cheese, Neufchâtel	75	259	22
Cheese, Parmesan	1,140	393	26
Cheese, provolone	764	350	25
Cheese, romano	1,078	385	25
Cheese, ricotta (part skim)	295	149	9
Cheese, ricotta (whole milk)	207	189	13
Cheese, Swiss	925	370	28
Cherries	19	70	0
Chestnuts*	17	194	2
Chicken, roasted	10	290	20
Chickpeas (garbanzos)	150	360	5
Chili con carne, with beans	32	133	6
Chili con carne, without beans	38	200	15
Chives	69	28	0
Chocolate milk, 3.5% fat	194	204	4
Chop suey, with meat	35	62	3
Chow mein, chicken	23	102	4
Clams, canned	55	52	1
Clams, raw	69	80	1
Coconut	− 37	346	35
Cod	10	78	0
Coffee, cup, regular	− 10	0	0
Coleslaw, with mayonnaise	44	144	14
Cookies, assorted	37	480	20
Corn, sweet	1	96	1
Cornflakes	8	386	0
Cowpeas (blackeyed peas)*	24	108	1
Crab, canned	45	101	3

Food	True calcium available mg per 100 g	Calories	% fat
Crab, deviled	47	188	9
Crab, steamed	43	93	2
Crackers, animal	52	429	9
Crackers, graham, plain	40	384	9
Crackers, saltines	21	433	12
Crackers, soda	22	439	13
Cranberries*	14	46	1
Cranberry juice cocktail*	5	65	0
Cranberry sauce, sweetened*	6	146	0
Crayfish	77	72	1
Cream puffs with custard	81	233	14
Cream, half-and-half	108	134	12
Cream, light whipping	85	300	31
Cucumbers	25	15	0
Currants, black, European*	58	54	0
Currants, red and white*	28	50	0
Custard, baked	112	115	6
Dates*	59	274	1
Doughnuts, cake-type	40	391	19
Duck	10	326	29
Eclair	80	239	14
Eel, American	18	233	18
Egg	54	163	12
Eggplant	8	25	0
Elderberries*	38	72	1
Endive and escarole	80	20	0
Fennel, leaves	98	28	0
Figs, dried*	126	274	1
Figs, fresh*	35	80	0
Flounder, baked	23	202	8
Frog legs	18	73	0
Fruit cocktail	9	76	0
Garlic, clove	27	137	0
Ginger root*	23	49	1
Goose, roasted	11	426	36
Gooseberries	−6	39	0
Grapefruit, all types	15	41	0
Grapefruit juice, all types	9	39	0
Grape juice, bottled	9	66	0

Food	True calcium available mg per 100 g	Calories	% fat
Grapes, Thompson	5	67	0
Guavas*	23	62	1
Haddock, fried	40	165	6
Halibut, broiled	16	171	7
Ham croquette	69	251	15
Ham, medium fat, roasted	10	374	31
Herring, canned	147	208	14
Honey	5	304	0
Horseradish (1 ounce)	40	87	0
Ice cream (10% fat)	146	193	11
Jams and preserves	20	272	0
Jellies	21	273	0
Kale	176	38	1
Kidneys, beef, braised	17	252	12
Kohlrabi*	40	29	0
Kumquats*	63	65	0
Lake herring (cisco)	12	96	2
Lamb, leg, roasted	10	279	19
Lard	0	902	100
Leeks	32	52	0
Lemon juice	6	25	0
Lemons, peeled fruit	26	27	0
Lentils, dry	− 14	340	1
Lettuce, butterhead	35	14	0
Lime juice*	9	26	0
Limes*	33	28	0
Liquor, hard (1.5 ounces)	− 15	263	0
Liver, beef, fried	9	229	11
Lobster Newburg	87	194	11
Lobster salad	36	110	6
Lobster, northern	65	95	2
Loganberries*	35	62	1
Loquats*	20	48	0
Lychees*	8	64	0
Macaroni and cheese	83	95	4
Macaroni, cooked	10	148	1
Mackerel, Atlantic, raw	5	191	12
Mackerel, Pacific	8	159	7
Mangos*	10	66	0

Food	True calcium available mg per 100 g	Calories	% fat
Maple syrup*	104	252	1
Margarine	20	720	81
Marmalade, citrus	32	257	0
Milk, butter (8 ounces)	277	82	0
Milk, evaporated	252	137	8
Milk, low-fat (2%) (8 ounces)	273	125	2
Milk, nonfat (8 ounces)	277	90	0
Milk, whole, 3.5% fat (8 ounces)	270	160	4
Muffins, plain	104	294	10
Mushrooms	5	28	0
Mussels	88	95	2
Mustard greens	183	31	1
Mustard, prepared (½ ounce)	18	91	6
Nectarines*	4	64	0
Noodles, egg	10	125	2
Oatmeal, cooked	− 17	55	1
Ocean perch	20	88	1
Octopus	29	73	1
Oil, cooking	0	884	100
Okra	26	36	0
Olives*	61	116	13
Onions*	25	38	0
Orange juice	10	48	0
Oranges	38	49	0
Oysters	94	66	2
Pancakes	101	231	7
Papayas*	20	39	0
Parsley	164	44	1
Parsnips	30	76	1
Passion fruit (Granadilla)*	13	90	1
Peaches	9	38	0
Peanut butter	− 163	581	49
Peanuts, roasted	− 163	581	49
Pears	5	61	0
Peas, boiled	22	43	0
Peas, green, baby, boiled	18	71	0
Pecans	− 19	687	71
Peppers, chili, green	6	37	0

Food	True calcium available mg per 100 g	Calories	% fat
Persimmons, raw	27	127	0
Pickles, cucumbers, dill	26	11	0
Pickles, relish, sweet	20	138	1
Pie, apple	8	256	11
Pie, banana custard	66	221	9
Pineapple, fresh*	17	52	0
Pineapple, heavy syrup*	10	74	0
Pineapple juice*	15	55	0
Pizza, with cheese	156	245	7
Plums, Damson*	13	66	0
Pomegranate*	3	63	0
Popcorn, oil and salt added	8	456	22
Pork, loin, broiled	11	391	32
Potato chips	20	568	40
Potatoes, baked	9	93	0
Potatoes, boiled	2	76	0
Pretzels	22	390	5
Prune juice, bottled*	14	77	0
Prunes*	48	255	1
Pumpkin*	25	33	0
Radishes*	30	17	0
Raisins*	62	289	0
Raspberries, black	26	73	1
Rhubarb	− 148	16	0
Rhubarb, cooked, with sugar	− 125	141	0
Rice pudding with raisins*	98	146	3
Rice, white, cooked	− 1	109	0
Roe, cod or shad, baked	13	126	3
Rolls, plain (pan rolls)	74	298	6
Roseapples*	29	56	0
Rusk*	20	419	9
Rutabagas, boiled	55	35	0
Salad dressing, blue cheese	81	504	52
Salad dressing, French	11	410	39
Salad dressing, Italian	10	552	60
Salad dressing, Mayonnaise	18	718	80
Salad dressing, Russian	19	494	51
Salad dressing, thousand island	11	502	50

Food	True calcium available mg per 100 g	Calories	% fat
Salmon, Atlantic	79	217	13
Salmon, Pacific	220	163	9
Sapodilla*	21	89	1
Sapotes (marmalade plums)*	39	125	1
Sardines, in oil	354	311	24
Sardines, in tomato sauce	448	197	12
Sauerkraut, canned*	36	18	0
Scallops, bay or sea, steamed	115	112	1
Shallots	37	72	0
Shrimp	215	106	2
Soybeans, boiled	73	130	6
Spaghetti, cooked	10	148	1
Spinach	−166	23	0
Squash, summer, boiled	15	14	0
Strawberries	16	37	1
Sugar, white, granulated	0	385	0
Sweet potatoes, baked	14	141	1
Swordfish	19	174	6
Swordfish, broiled	27	118	4
Tangerine juice*	18	43	0
Tangerines*	40	46	0
Tea, steeped 2 minutes (8-ounce cup)	−20	2	0
Tea, steeped 4 minutes (8-ounce cup)	−40	2	0
Tea, steeped 6 minutes (8-ounce cup)	−60	2	0
Tofu, firm	159	87	5
Tofu, soft	94	53	3
Tomato juice	5	19	0
Tomato puree*	13	39	0
Tomatoes, raw	12	22	0
Turnips	34	23	0
Walnuts	−59	651	64
Watercress	146	19	0
Watermelon*	7	26	0
Wheat germ	−50	363	11
Wheat, shredded	−157	354	2
Whitefish, lake	22	155	7

Food	True calcium available mg per 100 g	Calories	% fat
Wine, 12.2% alcohol	8	85	0
Yams, raw	20	101	0
Yogurt, fruit, low-fat (8 ounces)	305	204	1
Yogurt, plain, low-fat (8 ounces)	411	119	1

Note for professionals: This calcium counter is an educational tool to help in selection of foods that will maximize absorption of calcium. There are two common compounds in foods that interfere with calcium absorption: phytic acid and oxalic acid. A group of scientists, including Dr. June L. Kelsay of the nutritional research center of the U.S. Department of Agriculture and Dr. John W. Erdman, Jr. of the University of Illinois at Urbana, have been studying the effects of these acids on calcium absorption. They have provided valuable advice used in computation of this table.

We have generally assumed that one mole of oxalic acid binds one mole of calcium, and one mole of phytic acid binds three moles of calcium. These assumptions are supported by several clinical studies of unadapted individuals.

Exposure to compounds that bind calcium tends to be episodic in individuals consuming a varied Western diet, so there is relatively little opportunity for adaptation over the long term. Adaptation may also be limited at the low levels of calcium intake present in much of the U.S. population.

*Foods marked with an asterisk have not been fully analyzed for phytate and/or oxalate content in the open literature, and the true calcium content is our best estimate from available data.

Appendix B

Drinking Water In Major U.S. Cities

Instructions: Content of each mineral is shown by state and city. The most healthful waters have high levels of calcium (over 40 milligrams per liter) and magnesium (over 15 milligrams per liter) and low levels of sodium (less than 50 milligrams per liter).

State/City	Average calcium (milligrams per liter)	Average magnesium (milligrams per liter)	Average sodium (milligrams per liter)
Alabama			
Birmingham	27	5	9
Mobile	10	0	3
Montgomery	11	1	54
Alaska			
Anchorage	0	0	0
Arizona			
Mesa	0	0	0
Phoenix	39	15	63
Tucson	61	8	44
Arkansas			
Little Rock	0	0	0

State/City	Average calcium (milligrams per liter)	Average magnesium (milligrams per liter)	Average sodium (milligrams per liter)
California			
Anaheim	0	0	0
Fresno	15	11	17
Huntington Beach	0	0	0
Long Beach	26	5	124
Los Angeles	42	12	68
Oakland	8	1	3
Riverside	0	0	0
Sacramento	15	6	10
San Diego	40	16	57
San Francisco	8	2	5
San Jose	41	14	23
Santa Ana	0	0	0
Stockton	0	0	0
Colorado			
Aurora	0	0	0
Colorado Springs	0	0	0
Denver	17	5	13
District of Columbia			
Washington	39	9	9
Florida			
Jacksonville	65	23	14
Miami	21	3	17
St. Petersburg	33	3	6
Tampa	50	5	8
Georgia			
Atlanta	8	1	2
Columbus	0	0	0
Hawaii			
Honolulu	3	6	24
Illinois			
Chicago	33	11	4
Indiana			
Fort Wayne	28	4	15
Indianapolis	69	24	11
Iowa			
Des Moines	11	14	25

State/City	Average calcium (milligrams per liter)	Average magnesium (milligrams per liter)	Average sodium (milligrams per liter)
Kansas			
Kansas City	57	11	25
Wichita	22	9	61
Kentucky			
Lexington	0	0	0
Louisville	24	10	26
Louisiana			
Baton Rouge	1	0	66
New Orleans	20	8	18
Shreveport	19	4	24
Maryland			
Baltimore	25	5	6
Massachusetts			
Boston	5	0	2
Worcester	4	0	3
Michigan			
Detroit	28	7	4
Grand Rapids	34	11	5
Warren	0	0	0
Minnesota			
Minneapolis	18	5	7
St. Paul	23	1	5
Mississippi			
Jackson	16	1	3
Missouri			
Kansas City	20	5	38
St. Louis	22	6	22
Nebraska			
Lincoln	56	9	25
Omaha	35	14	65
Nevada			
Las Vegas	0	0	0
New Jersey			
Jersey City	11	4	5
Newark	11	3	4
New Mexico			
Albuquerque	30	4	37

State/City	Average calcium (milligrams per liter)	Average magnesium (milligrams per liter)	Average sodium (milligrams per liter)
New York			
Buffalo	38	9	9
New York	9	2	3
Rochester	28	6	6
Syracuse	35	6	2
Yonkers	14	5	8
North Carolina			
Charlotte	9	2	4
Greensboro	21	2	3
Ohio			
Akron	35	7	6
Cincinnati	45	10	18
Cleveland	35	7	11
Columbus	32	5	19
Dayton	27	10	17
Toledo	19	5	12
Oklahoma			
Oklahoma City	29	16	84
Tulsa	31	2	4
Oregon			
Portland	1	1	1
Pennsylvania			
Philadelphia	25	5	6
Pittsburgh	20	5	11
Tennessee			
Chattanooga	28	5	8
Knoxville	0	0	0
Memphis	8	4	10
Nashville	25	4	4
Texas			
Arlington	0	0	0
Austin	17	16	33
Corpus Christi	42	8	62
Dallas	23	4	38
El Paso	13	4	63
Fort Worth	45	8	20
Houston	13	2	34

State/City	Average calcium (milligrams per liter)	Average magnesium (milligrams per liter)	Average sodium (milligrams per liter)
Lubbock	53	20	36
San Antonio	0	0	0
Utah			
Salt Lake City	32	8	6
Virginia			
Norfolk	21	3	9
Richmond	16	3	4
Virginia Beach	0	0	0
Washington			
Seattle	7	1	2
Spokane	26	12	2
Tacoma	4	1	3
Wisconsin			
Madison	43	27	3
Milwaukee	35	10	4

Appendix C

Calcium, Calories, and Fat Content of Some Popular Fast Foods

Food	Calcium mg per svg	Calories per svg	Calcium/ Calorie Ratio	Fat (g) per svg	% Calories as Fat
Burger King					
Salad with reduced calorie Italian dressing	40	42	0.95	0	0
Onion Rings, Regular	124	274	0.45	16	53
Ham and Cheese Sandwich	195	471	0.41	23	44
Breakfast Croissan'wich with Ham, Egg, Cheese	136	335	0.41	20	54

Food	Calcium mg per svg	Calories per svg	Calcium/ Calorie Ratio	Fat (g) per svg	% Calories as Fat
Breakfast Croissan'wich with Bacon, Egg, Cheese	136	355	0.38	24	61
Salad with Bleu Cheese Dressing	66	184	0.36	16	78
Bacon Double Cheeseburger	168	510	0.33	31	55
Cheeseburger	102	317	0.32	15	43
Whopper with Cheese	215	711	0.30	43	54
Salad with 1000 Island Dressing	42	145	0.29	12	74
Whopper Jr. with Cheese	105	364	0.29	20	49
Salad with House Dressing	44	158	0.28	13	74
Breakfast Croissan'wich with Sausage, Egg, Cheese	145	538	0.27	41	69
Scrambled Egg Platter	101	468	0.22	30	58
Scrambled Egg with Bacon	103	536	0.19	36	60
Great Danish	91	500	0.18	36	65
Scrambled Egg with Sausage	112	702	0.16	52	67
French Toast Sticks	77	499	0.15	29	52
Hamburger	37	275	0.13	12	39
Whopper Sandwich	84	628	0.13	36	52
Whopper Junior	40	322	0.12	17	48
Chicken Sandwich	79	688	0.11	40	52
Whaler Sandwich	46	488	0.09	27	50
Chicken Tenders (6)	18	204	0.09	10	44

Food	Calcium mg per svg	Calories per svg	Calcium/ Calorie Ratio	Fat (g) per svg	% Calories as Fat
Kentucky Fried Chicken					
Baked Beans	54	105	0.51	1	9
Mashed Potatoes	21	59	0.36	1	15
Mashed Potatoes with Gravy	19	62	0.31	1	15
Buttermilk Biscuit (one)	77	269	0.29	14	47
Cole Slaw	29	103	0.28	6	52
Original Recipe Wing	38	181	0.21	12	60
Original Recipe Side Breast	48	276	0.17	17	55
Chicken Gravy	9	59	0.15	4	61
Original Recipe Center Breast	39	257	0.15	14	49
Extra Crispy Thigh	46	371	0.12	26	63
Original Recipe Thigh	28	278	0.10	19	62
Extra Crispy Center Breast	35	353	0.10	21	54
Extra Crispy Wing	21	218	0.10	16	66
Extra Crispy Side Breast	32	354	0.09	24	61
Kentucky Fries	24	268	0.09	13	44
Original Recipe Drumstick	13	147	0.09	9	55
Extra Crispy Drumstick	15	173	0.09	11	57
Potato Salad	11	141	0.08	9	57
Kentucky Nugget (one)	2	46	0.04	3	59
Corn-on-the-Cob	7	176	0.04	3	15
McDonald's					
Soft Serve Cone	183	189	0.97	5	24

Food	Calcium mg per svg	Calories per svg	Calcium/ Calorie Ratio	Fat (g) per svg	% Calories as Fat
Vanilla Milk Shake	329	352	0.93	8	20
Strawberry Milk Shake	322	362	0.89	9	22
Chocolate Milk Shake	320	383	0.84	9	21
Egg McMuffin	226	340	0.66	16	42
English Muffin with Butter	117	186	0.63	5	24
Hot Fudge Sundae	215	367	0.59	11	27
Hot Caramel Sundae	200	361	0.55	10	25
Strawberry Sundae	174	320	0.54	9	25
Cheeseburger	169	318	0.53	16	45
Quarter Pounder with Cheese	255	525	0.49	32	55
Sausage McMuffin	168	427	0.39	26	55
Sausage McMuffin with Egg	196	517	0.38	33	57
McD.L.T.	250	680	0.37	44	58
Big Mac	203	570	0.36	35	55
Scrambled Eggs	61	180	0.34	13	65
Hamburger	84	263	0.32	11	38
Filet-O-Fish	133	435	0.31	26	54
Quarter Pounder	98	427	0.23	24	51
Biscuit with Biscuit Spread	74	330	0.22	18	49
Hotcakes with Butter, Syrup	103	500	0.21	10	18
Biscuit with Sausage, Egg	119	585	0.20	40	62
Biscuit with Sausage	82	467	0.18	31	60
Chocolaty Chip Cookies	29	342	0.08	16	42

Food	Calcium mg per svg	Calories per svg	Calcium/ Calorie Ratio	Fat (g) per svg	% Calories as Fat
Iced Cheese Danish	33	395	0.08	22	50
Cinnamon Raisin Danish	35	445	0.08	21	42
Pork Sausage	16	210	0.08	19	81
Apple Pie	14	253	0.06	14	50
French Fries	9	220	0.04	12	49
McDonaldland Cookies	12	308	0.04	11	32
Apple Danish	14	389	0.04	18	42
Hashbrown Potatoes	5	144	0.03	9	56
Chicken McNuggets	11	323	0.03	20	56
Raspberry Danish	14	414	0.03	16	35
Wendy's					
Mozzarella Cheese (imitation)	160	90	1.78	7	70
Frosty Dairy Dessert	240	400	0.60	14	32
Taco Salad	240	430	0.56	19	40
Cheese Potato	280	590	0.47	34	52
Omelet #3	120	280	0.43	19	61
Broccoli & Cheese Potato	200	500	0.40	25	45
Chili & Cheese Potato	200	510	0.39	20	35
Breakfast Sandwich	120	370	0.32	19	46
Omelet #2	80	250	0.32	17	61
Bacon & Cheese Potato	160	570	0.28	30	47
Omelet #1	80	290	0.28	21	65
Scrambled Eggs	48	190	0.25	12	57
Buttermilk Biscuit	80	320	0.25	17	48
Omelet #4	48	210	0.23	15	64
White Bun	32	140	0.23	2	13

Food	Calcium mg per svg	Calories per svg	Calcium/ Calorie Ratio	Fat (g) per svg	% Calories as Fat
Chili	48	240	0.20	8	30
Fried Egg	16	90	0.18	6	60
French Toast	64	400	0.16	19	43
Kids' Hamburger	32	200	0.16	9	41
Cheese Danish	64	430	0.15	21	44
Cinnamon Raisin Danish	48	410	0.12	18	40
Kaiser Bun	16	180	0.09	2	10
Chicken Fried Steak	48	580	0.08	41	64
Sausage Gravy	32	440	0.07	36	74
Sour Cream & Chives Potato	32	460	0.07	24	47
Big Classic	32	470	0.07	25	48
White Toast with Margarine	16	250	0.06	9	32
Crispy Cook'n Nuggets (in animal/vegetable oil)	16	290	0.06	21	65
Crispy Cook'n Nuggets (in vegetable oil)	16	310	0.05	21	61
Breakfast Potatoes	16	360	0.04	22	55

Appendix D

Calcium, Calories, and Fat Content of Some Popular Prepared Foods

Food	Calcium mg per svg	Calories per svg	Calcium/ Calorie Ratio	Fat (g) per svg	% Calories as Fat
Armour Dinner Classics					
Seafood Newburg	100	300	0.33	12	36
Chicken Fricassee	100	340	0.29	11	29
Veal Parmagiana	100	400	0.25	22	50
Chicken and Noodles	80	340	0.24	13	34
Chicken with Wine, Mushroom Sauce	80	350	0.23	18	46
Turkey and Dressing	60	330	0.18	14	38
Salisbury Steak	60	460	0.13	25	49
Yankee Pot Roast	40	390	0.10	17	39

Food	Calcium mg per svg	Calories per svg	Calcium/ Calorie Ratio	Fat (g) per svg	% Calories as Fat
Birdseye Fresh Creations					
Tortellini & Broccoli					
Sauterne	500	520	0.96	24	42
Chicken in Swiss					
Mornay	200	330	0.61	13	35
Pasta Primavera	200	620	0.32	22	32
Chicken Oriental	40	270	0.15	3	10
Beef Oriental	60	440	0.14	13	27
Campbell Soup Le Menu					
Lite Style Beef à					
l'Orange	80	290	0.28	7	22
Chicken Cordon					
Bleu	100	460	0.22	19	37
Beef Sirloin Tips					
with Gravy	80	390	0.21	22	51
Ham Steak	48	320	0.15	10	28
Sliced Turkey Breast with Potatoes, Broccoli Gravy, Rice, Vegetables	40	460	0.09	30	59
Stouffer's Lean Cuisine					
Cheese Cannelloni with Tomato Sauce	300	270	1.11	10	33
Tuna Lasagna	250	280	0.89	10	32
Chicken & Vegetables with Vermicelli	100	270	0.37	7	23
Turkey Dijon	100	280	0.36	11	35
Oriental Scallops & Vegetables with Rice	60	220	0.27	3	12
Spaghetti with Beef, Mushroom Sauce	60	280	0.21	7	23
Meatball Stew	40	250	0.16	10	36
Zucchini Lasagna	30	260	0.12	7	24

Food	Calcium mg per svg	Calories per svg	Calcium/ Calorie Ratio	Fat (g) per svg	% Calories as Fat
Chicken Chow Mein with Rice	20	250	0.08	5	18
Linguini with Clam Sauce	20	260	0.08	7	24
Weight Watchers					
Fillet of Fish Au Gratin	150	210	0.71	7	30
Breaded Chicken Patty Parmesan	150	290	0.52	18	56
Candle Lite Stuffed Sole with Potatoes, Broccoli	100	280	0.36	7	23
Oven Fried Fish	40	220	0.18	12	49
Southern Fried Chicken Patty	20	270	0.07	18	60

Appendix E
Oxalates in Foods

Instructions: Milligrams of oxalates per 3.5 ounce serving are shown below. Oxalates bind calcium, making it unavailable. In predisposed individuals, oxalates increase the risk of kidney stones. Individuals with a personal or family history of kidney stones should not consume more than 50 milligrams of oxalate per day.

Food	*Oxalate (mg/3.5 ounces)*
Spinach	750–1760
Rhubarb	860
Beets	675
Swiss chard	645
Wheat germ	270
Pecans	200
Peanuts	190
Parsley	165
Peppers, green and red	145
Okra	145
Chocolate (candy)	120
Lime peel	110
Leeks	90
Gooseberries	90
Lemon peel	85
Watercress	85

Food	Oxalate (mg/3.5 ounces)
Tea, black—steeped 6 min.	80
Tea, black—steeped 4 min.	70
Tea, black—steeped 2 min.	55
Tea, Darjeeling—steeped 1 min.	25
Tea, green—steeped 3 min.	35
Collards	75
Sweet potatoes	55
Raspberries, black	55
Cabbage, Chinese	50
Celery	25–50
Beans, green	45
Grits, corn	40
Eggplant	40
Hot cocoa (cup)	30
Carrots	6–30
Escarole	30
Grapes, Concord	25
Dandelion greens	25
Summer squash	20
Bread, whole wheat	20
Beans in tomato sauce	20
Currants, red	10–20
Rutabagas	20
Blackberries	20
Blueberries	15
Raspberries, red	15
Strawberries	15
Cauliflower	1–15
Dewberries	15
Kale	7–15
Fruit salad	10
Plums	0–10
Marmalade	10
Tomatoes	2–10
Parsnips	10

Food	*Oxalate (mg/3.5 ounces)*
Onions, green	10
Beansprouts (soy)	10
Strawberry jam	9
Artichokes	9
Cabbage	0–8
Mustard greens	8
Cake, sponge	7
Liver	7
Bread, white	7
Apricots	3–7
Cranberry juice	7
Oranges	4–6
Brussels sprouts	0–6
Lettuce	2–6
Grape juice	6
Prunes	6
Asparagus	2–5
Corn	5
Potatoes, white (boiled)	0–5
Cornflakes	5
Fennel	5
Garlic	5
Peaches	1–5
Tomato juice	5
Vegetable soup	5
Sardines	2–5
Currants, black	4
Lima beans	4
Beer	0–4
Rosehip tea	4
Spaghetti in tomato sauce	4

Food	Oxalate (mg/3.5 ounces)
Tofu, Mori-Nu (soft or firm)	4
Bacon (fried)	3
Grapefruit	3
Coffee (brewed)	2–3
Kidney, braised	3
Wine (Beaujolais)	3
Apples	2–3
Pears	2–3
Tomato soup	3
Kohlrabi	3
Endive	2
Mushrooms	2
Pork (roast)	2
Beef (roast)	0–2
Ham	1–2
Lamb (roast)	trace–2
Lemon juice	2
Pasta (boiled)	2
Pineapple (canned)	2
Wine (rose)	2
Orange juice	1
Cherries	1
Chicken (roast)	1
Chives	1
Coffee, instant	1
Peas	1
Chicken noodle soup	1
Chow mein noodles	1
Cucumber	1
Oatmeal (cooked)	1
Oxtail soup	1
Turnips (boiled)	1
Banana	1

Food	Oxalate (mg/3.5 ounces)
Milk	1
Plum jam, red	1
Pumpkin	1
Eggs (boiled)	1
Flounder (boiled)	1
Radishes	0–1
Beef, corned (canned)	0–1
Haddock	1
Apple juice	trace
Broccoli	trace
Coca-Cola	trace
Pepsi-Cola	trace
Sherry (dry)	trace
Wine (port)	trace
Avocado	0
Butter	0
Cantaloupe	0
Casaba melon	0
Cheese, cheddar	0
Cider	0
Grapes, Thompson	0
Grapefruit juice	0
Hamburger	0
Honeydew melon	0
Lime juice	0
Mangoes	0
Margarine	0
Nectarines	0
Onions, mature	0
Pineapple juice	0
Sugar candies	0
Rice (boiled)	0
Watermelon	0
Whortleberries, red	0
Wine (white)	0

References:

Ney D.M., et al. *The Low Oxalate Diet Book for the Prevention of Oxalate Kidney Stones*. San Diego: University of California at San Diego Medical Center, 1981.

Yamanaka H, et al. Determination of oxalate in foods by enzymatic analysis. *Journal of the Food Hygiene Society of Japan* 1983;24:454–458.

Ohkawa H. Gas chromatographic determination of oxalic acid in foods. *Journal of the Association of Official Analytical Chemists* 1985;68:108–11.

Kim EH and Im KJ. A study of oxalic acid and calcium content in Korean foods. *Korean Journal of Nutrition* 1977;10:292–298.

Hodgkinson A. *Oxalic Acid in Biology and Medicine*. New York: Academic Press, 1977.

Morinaga Milk Co., Ltd. Tokyo, Japan. Personal communication.

Lentner C., ed.: *Geigy Scientific Tables*, Vol 1, 8th ed. West Caldwell, NJ: Medical Education Division, Ciba-Geigy Corp., 1981.

Appendix F
Sources of Potassium

Food (3.5 oz portion, unless otherwise stated)	Potassium (mg)
Prunes, raw	940
Raisins, raw	763
Banana (1)	740
Figs, dried	640
Nectarine (1)	588
Sole, baked	587
Scallops, steamed	476
Mushrooms, raw	414
Turkey breast, roasted	411
Chicken breast, roasted	411
Potato, boiled in skin	407
Peach (1)	404
Broccoli, raw	382
Tomato (1)	366
Salmon, canned sockeye	361
Celery, raw	341
Beets, raw	335
Milk, nonfat (8-oz glass)	334
Sardines, canned Pacific, drained	320
Clams, raw	311
Orange (1)	300
Plums, Damson (3)	299

Food (3.5 oz portion, unless otherwise stated)	Potassium (mg)
Cauliflower	295
Albacore tuna, raw	293
Apricot, raw	281
Asparagus, raw	278
Grapefruit (½)	270
Turnips, raw	268
Lettuce, butterhead	264
Cabbage, raw	233
Corn on the cob	196
Thompson grapes	173
Apple, raw (1)	165
Cucumber	160
Raisin roll (1)	147
Pineapple, raw	146
Ricotta	136
Shrimp, canned, drained	122
Swiss cheese	104
Cottage cheese	85
Blueberries, raw	81
Pasta	79

References and Bibliography

Ackley, S., E. Barrett-Connor, and L. Suarez. "Dairy products, calcium, and blood pressure." *American Journal of Clinical Nutrition* 38 (1983): 457–461.

Blot, W. J., et al. "Geographic patterns of large bowel cancer in the United States." *Journal of the National Cancer Institute* 57 (1976): 1125–31.

———"Geographic patterns of breast cancer in the United States." *Journal of the National Cancer Institute* 59 (1977): 1407–11.

Bouillon, R. A., et al. "Vitamin D status in the elderly: seasonal substrate deficiency causes 1,25-dihydroxycholecalciferol deficiency." *American Journal of Clinical Nutrition* 45 (1987): 755–63.

Buset, M., et al. "Inhibition of human colonic epithelial cell proliferation in vivo and in vitro by calcium." *Cancer Research* 46 (1986): 5426–30.

Canada, Minister of National Health and Welfare. *Mortality Atlas of Canada.* Hull, Quebec: Canadian Government Publishing Centre, 1980: Map 17.

Charlson, R. J., et al. "The dominance of tropospheric sulfate in modifying solar radiation." In *Radiation in the Atmosphere,* ed. H. J. Bolle. Princeton: Science Press, 1977: 32–38.

Colston, K., J. R. Wilkinson, and R. C. Coombes. "1,25-dihydroxyvitamin D_3 binding in estrogen-responsive rat breast tumor." *Endocrinology* 119 (1986): 397–403.

Cummings, S. R. et al. "Epidemiology of osteoporosis and osteoporotic fractures." *Epidemiologic Reviews* 7 (1985): 178–208.

Facchini, U., et al. "Geographical variation of cancer mortality in Italy." *International Journal of Epidemiology* 14 (1985): 538–48.

Gardner, M. J., et al. *Atlas of Cancer Mortality in England and Wales, 1968–1978.* Chichester, U.K.: John Wiley and Sons, 1983.

Garland, C. F., et al. "Dietary vitamin D and calcium and risk of colorect cancer: a nineteen-year prospective study in men." *Lancet* 1 (1985): 307–9.

Garland, C. F., and F. C. Garland. "Calcium and colon cancer." *Clinical Nutrition* 5 (1986): 161–66.

——"Do sunlight and vitamin D reduce the likelihood of colon cancer?" *International Journal of Epidemiology* 9 (1980): 227–31.

Garn, S. M., and V. M. Hawthorne. "Calcium intake and bone loss in population context." In: *Calcium in Biological Systems.* ed. R. P. Rubin, G. B. Weiss, and J. W. Putney, Jr. New York: Plenum Press, 1985: 569–74.

Greenberg, M. R. *Urbanization and Cancer Mortality: The United States Experience, 1950–1975.* Monographs in epidemiology and biostatistics, volume 4. New York: Oxford University Press, 1983.

Grinstead, C. W., C. Y. C. Pak, and G. J. Krejs. "Effect of 1,25-dihydroxyvitamin D_3 on calcium absorption in the colon of healthy humans." *American Journal of Physiology* 247 (1984): G189–92.

Hall, F. M., M. A. Davis, and D. T. Baran. "Bone mineral screening of osteoporosis." *New England Journal of Medicine* 316 (1987): 212–14.

Haussler, M. R. "Vitamin D receptors: nature and function." *Annual Review of Nutrition* 6 (1986): 527–62.

Heaney, R. P., and R. R. Recker. "Distribution of calcium absorption in middle-aged women." *American Journal of Clinical Nutrition* 43 (1986): 299–305.

Hidy, G. M. *Aerosols.* New York: Academic Press 1984.

Hodgkinson, A. *Oxalic Acid in Biology and Medicine.* New York: Academic Press, 1977.

Holick, M. F., J. A. MacLaughlin, and S. H. Doppelt. "Regulation of cutaneous previtamin D_3 photosynthesis in man: skin pigment is not an essential regulator." *Science* 211 (1981): 590–93.

Karanja, N., and D. A. McCarron. "Calcium and hypertension." *Annual Review of Nutrition* 6 (1986): 475–94.

Kelsay, J. L. "Effect of oxalic acid on calcium bioavailability." In *Nutritional bioavailability of calcium,* ed. C. Kies. Based on a symposium sponsored by the Division of Agricultural and Food Chemistry at the 187th Meeting of the American Chemical Society, St. Louis, Missouri April 8–13, 1984. ACS Symposium Series 275. Washington, D.C.: American Chemical Society, 1985: 105–16.

Krueger, A. J. "Sighting of El Chichon sulfur dioxide clouds with the

Nimbus 7 total ozone mapping spectrometer." *Science* 220 (1983): 1377–79.

Kolonel, L. N. "Fat and colon cancer: How firm is the epidemiologic evidence?" *American Journal of Clinical Nutrition* 45 (1987): 336–41.

Kondrat'ev K. Y. A. *Radiation Characteristics of the Atmosphere and the Earth's Surface.* (Translated from the Russian.) New Delhi: Amerind Publishing Co., 1973.

Landsberg, H. E., et al. *World Maps of Climatology,* 2nd ed. New York: Springer-Verlag, 1965.

Lilienfeld, A. M., and D. E. Lilienfeld. *Foundations of Epidemiology,* 2nd ed. New York: Oxford University Press, 1980.

Lipkin, M., and H. Newmark. "Effect of added dietary calcium on colonic epithelial-cell proliferation in subjects at high risk for familial colonic cancer." *New England Journal of Medicine* 313 (1985): 1381–84.

London, J. "The depletion of ultraviolet radiation by atmospheric ozone." In *The Biologic Effects of Ultraviolet Radiation (with Emphasis on the Skin).* ed F. Urbach. New York: Pergamon Press, 1969: 335–39.

McCance, R. A., and E. M. Widdowson. "Mineral metabolism of healthy adults on white and brown bread dietaries." *Journal of Physiology* (London) (1942–43): 44.

McCarron, D. A., and C. D. Morris. "Blood pressure response to oral calcium in persons with mild to moderate hypertension." *Annals of Internal Medicine* 103 (1985): 825–31.

MacLaughlin, J. A., R. R. Anderson, and M. F. Holick. "Spectral character of sunlight modulates photosynthesis of previtamin D_3 and its photoisomers in human skin." *Science* 216 (1982): 1001–3.

Martin, C. J., and W. J. Evans. "Phytic acid–metal ion interactions. I. The effect of pH on CA(II) binding." *Journal of Inorganic Biochemistry* 27 (1986) 17–30.

Mason, T. J., et al. *Atlas of Cancer Mortality for U.S. Counties: 1950–69.* DHEW Publication No. (NIH) 75-780. Washington, D.C.: U.S. Government Printing Office, 1975.

Matkovic, V., et al. "Bone status and fracture rates in two regions of Yugoslavia." *American Journal of Clinical Nutrition* 32 (1979): 540–49.

Miyaura, C., et al. "1,25-dihydroxyvitamin D_3 induces differentiation of human myeloid leukemia cells." *Biochemical and Biophysical Research Communications* 102 (1981): 937–43.

Modan, B., et al. "Low-fiber intake as an etiologic factor in cancer of the colon." *Journal of the National Cancer Institute* 55 (1975): 15–18.

Napalkov, N. P., et al. *Cancer Incidence in the USSR.* Supplement to *Cancer Incidence in Five Continents,* Volume 3. IARC Scientific Publication No. 48. Lyon: International Agency for Research on Cancer, 1983: 59.

Newmark, H. L., M. J. Wargovich, and W. R. Bruce. "Colon cancer and dietary fat, phosphate, and calcium: A hypothesis." *Journal of the National Cancer Institute* 72 (1984): 1323–25.

Ney, D. M., et al. *The Low Oxalate Diet Book for the Prevention of Oxalate Kidney Stones.* San Diego: General Clinical Research Center, University of California, San Diego, 1981.

Palm, T. A. "The geographical distribution and aetiology of rickets." *The Practitioner* 45 (1890): 270–79.

Pennington, J. A. T., and H. N. Church. *Bowes and Church's Food Values of Portions Commonly Used,* 14th ed. Philadelphia: J.B. Lippincott Co., 1985.

Petrakis, N. L., V. L. Ernster, and M.-C. King. "Breast." In *Cancer Epidemiology and Prevention,* ed. D. Schottenfeld and J. F. Fraumeni, Jr. Philadelphia: W. B. Saunders Company, 1982: 855–70.

Phillips, R. L., and D. A. Snowdon. "Dietary relationships with fatal colorectal cancer among Seventh-Day Adventists." *Journal of the National Cancer Institute* 74 (1985): 307–17.

Potter, J. D., and A. J. McMichael. "Diet and cancer of the colon and rectum: A case-control study." *Journal of the National Cancer Institute* 76 (1986): 557–69.

Recker, R. R., and R. P. Heaney. "The effect of milk supplements on calcium metabolism, bone metabolism, and calcium balance." *American Journal of Clinical Nutrition* 41 (1985): 254–63.

Schottenfeld, D., and S. J. Winawer. "Large intestine." In *Cancer Epidemiology and Prevention,* ed. D. Schottenfeld and J. F. Fraumeni, Jr. Philadelphia: W.B. Saunders Company, 1982: 703–27.

Scotto, J., T. E. Fears, and J. F. Fraumeni, Jr. "Solar radiation." In *Cancer Epidemiology and Prevention,* ed. D. Schottenfeld and J. F. Fraumeni, Jr. Philadelphia: W.B. Saunders Company, 1982: 254–76.

Scotto, J., T. R. Fears, and G. B. Gori. "Ultraviolet exposure patterns, 1976." *Environmental Research* 12 (1976):228–37.

Seidman, H., and S. D. Stellman, "A different perspective on breast cancer risk: Some implications of the nonattributable risk." *Cancer* 32 (1982): 301–13.

Shekeller, R. B., et al. "Dietary vitamin A and risk of cancer in the Western Electric study." *Lancet* 2 (1981):1185–90.

Shimkin, M. B. *Science and Cancer,* 3rd rev. Washington, D.C.: U.S.

Department of Health and Human Services, National Cancer Institute, 1980.

Smith, L. H. "The diagnosis and treatment of metabolic stone disease." *Medical Clinics of North America* 56 (1972): 977–88.

Solomons, N. W. "Calcium intake and availability from the human diet." *Clinical Nutrition* 5 (1986): 167–76.

Sowers, M. R., et al. "The association of intakes of vitamin D and calcium with blood pressure among women." *American Journal of Clinical Nutrition* 42 (1985): 135–42.

Waggoner, A. P., et al. "Optical characteristics of atmospheric aerosols." *Atmospheric Environment* 15 (1981): 1891–1909.

Wargovich, M. J., V. W. Eng, and H. L. Newmark. "Calcium inhibits the damaging and compensatory proliferative effects of fatty acids on mouse colon epithelium." *Cancer Letters* 23 (1984): 253–58.

Warshauer, M. C., et al. "Stomach and colorectal cancers in Puerto Rican–born residents of New York City." *Journal of the National Cancer Institute* 75 (1986): 592–95.

Willett, W. C., et al. "Dietary fat and the risk of breast cancer." *New England Journal of Medicine* 316 (1987): 22–28.

INDEX